KEEPING YOUR FAMILY SAFE

THE RESPONSIBILITIES OF FIREARM OWNERSHIP

TIMOTHY W. WHEELER, MD

E. JOHN WIPFLER III, MD

Merril Press
Bellevue, Washington

Keeping Your Family Safe
Merril Press, P.O. Box 1682, Bellevue, WA 98009
www.merrilpress.com
Phone: 425-454-7008

Distributed to the book trade by
Midpoint Trade Books, 27 W. 20th Street,
New York, N.Y. 10011
www.midpointtradebooks.com
Phone: 212-727-0190

Library of Congress Cataloging-in-Publication Data

Wheeler, Timothy W.
    Keeping your family safe : the responsibilities of firearm ownership /
Timothy W. Wheeler, E. John Wipfler. -- 1st ed.
        p. cm.
    ISBN-13: 978-0-936783-56-7 (pbk.)
    ISBN-10: 0-936783-56-7 (pbk.)
    1. Firearms ownership--United States. 2. Home accidents--
Prevention. I. Wipfler, E. John. II. Title.
    HV8059.W48 2009
    623.4'420289--dc22
                                                2009022528

Printed in the United States of America

Keeping Your Family Safe

Doctors for Responsible Gun Ownership

A Project of The Claremont Institute

937 West Foothill Boulevard, Suite E
Claremont, California 91711

Telephone (909) 621-6825
Fax (909) 626-8724
www.claremont.org

About the Authors

Timothy W. Wheeler, MD is the director of Doctors for Responsible Gun Ownership (DRGO), a Project of the Claremont Institute. DRGO is a nationwide group of physicians, scientists, medical students, and others who support the safe and lawful use of firearms. Dr. Wheeler is a surgeon practicing in Ontario, California. He has taken training in the moral, ethical, legal, and tactical aspects of defensive firearm use at the Lethal Force Institute under Massad Ayoob. He has passed the Tactical Handgun course, Parts I and II at the Tactical Firearms Training Team. His editorial articles on firearm policy have appeared in the *Washington Times*, the *Miami Herald*, *National Review Online*, and others. His television appearances have included Fox News television, CBS *This Morning* and CBS News *60 Minutes*.

E. John Wipfler III, MD, FACEP is associate clinical professor at the University of Illinois College of Medicine and attending emergency physician at OSF Saint Francis Medical Center, a Level I trauma center in Peoria, Illinois. Dr. Wipfler is the Medical Director for an agency providing tactical emergency medicine support (TEMS) for three tactical law enforcement teams. He has been involved in over 80 SWAT callouts and serves as the Sheriff's Physician and sworn auxiliary deputy sheriff with the Peoria County Sheriff's Department. He co-chairs the TEMS committee with the Illinois Tactical Officer's Association and Illinois Department of Public Health. Dr. Wipfler has 14 years of military experience with the United States Army Reserve Medical Corps. He is a certified firearms safety instructor and has completed firearms training with the U.S. Army, Chapman Academy, InSights Training Center, Combat Casualty Care Course, CONTOMS, and the Heckler & Koch TEMS International Training Division. He is an instructor with the International School of Tactical Medicine.

Disclaimer

This book is intended to address firearms in a general way only. The authors are not legal experts, nor do we intend to give legal advice. As our book will make clear, the laws regarding the use of firearms for defense are extremely complex and quite variable from one state to another and even from one community to another. No single book can address them all.

Neither the authors nor the publisher can be responsible for the results of firearm use by a person relying only on our book. We strongly urge our readers to learn safe and responsible firearm use through training by qualified experts, but we cannot guarantee the results of such training.

Especially in preparing to use firearms for defense, we recommend training by an expert in the legal principles of the use of deadly force, as well as training in the use of the firearm itself. For any questions about the legality of deadly force we recommend that the reader consult a lawyer.

Advice regarding first aid should be considered general advice only. The authors cannot guarantee the medical outcome of any application of this advice in a particular medical situation,

CONTENTS

Foreword

For many, thoughts about guns and safety don't mix. Not only does the combination seem illogical to them, it arouses some degree of fright. In fact, there hasn't been such widespread and overblown fear since the hysteria of the Salem witch trials. Witches were believed to be evil and dangerous, a conviction that in its time was resistant to any consideration of fact. Today some believe that guns are evil or inordinately dangerous. That belief is just as irrational and just as immune to the facts. The fact is that gun owners have an outstanding safety record. There is an incontrovertible record of guns preventing death, injury and rape.

The belief that some people have of guns as evil and dangerous is evident everywhere. Media reports of crime, even those that don't involve guns, are typically highlighted with gun logos. In television coverage of police dogs sniffing for bombs, the camera pans to and focuses on the officer's firearm. Some branches of organized medicine lobby to ban guns or by incremental means to eliminate them. They publish biased research to assist in that effort. Such political activism is pursued in the name of public safety, but it actually has the opposite effect. The American colonial equivalent of organized medicine also practiced public safety during the witch trials. The supposed stigmata that proved a person to be a witch—so-called devil's marks—could only be diagnosed by physicians. Today, some guns are diagnosed as particularly evil because of their appearance.

The irrational fear of guns has many negative effects. The response to fear often results in denial and reaction formation. Some gun owners avoid proper training and practice or have too casual an attitude. They keep the gun as a talisman, thinking it will magically keep them safe. This thinking could lead to disaster if the gun were actually needed for defense. And too casual an attitude might cause a safety lapse. Reaction formation is a psychological defense against an unconscious impulse or fear. It causes opposite behavior. An example is when a person who fears heights seeks employment as a steeplejack. With guns, reaction formation is a defense against excessive unconscious fear of them. The gun owner employs false bravado in an attempt to subdue his unconscious fear.

Some people unduly fear their own normal aggressive impulses. Their excessive fear makes the idea of self-defense unacceptable to them. They might give the idea lip service—"of course I'd kill someone if they tried to rape my child!" However, they shun the use of guns or the training that would actually enable them to protect the child. The aforementioned hysteria, evident in political correctness, seeks to overly control normal aggressive impulses by outlawing bullying and even such innocent games as playing cowboys and Indians, and dodge ball.

Misplaced ethical concerns complicate these distorted reactions to guns, safety, and self-defense. One physician, trained in firearms and self-defense, was confronted with a hostage situation. A man had seized a woman and threatened her life. The doctor shot and killed the man, saving the woman's life and his own. But his medical society chastised the doctor. After all, they righteously insisted, physicians "should do no harm." Similarly, some people proclaim that killing, even in self-defense, is a sin. That's how they interpret the biblical admonition "Thou shall not kill." It is of course their right to give up their lives, or the lives of loved ones, to a vicious thug or societal misfit. Or is it? Not only do the major religions permit taking a life if necessary to save one, most say there is a moral duty to do so. In a chapter on ethics and the laws of self-defense, Dr. Wheeler touches on historical and philosophical perspectives. These viewpoints are vitally important reading to all who keep firearms for protection.

Equally important is the need for training and practice if one is serious about using a firearm for protection. Guns undoubtedly save more lives than do fire extinguishers. Schools and many institutions require training with fire extinguishers and periodic fire drills. Training and drills are even more important with that other safety-rescue device, the gun. Dr. Wipfler, in a chapter on firearms training, emphasizes the importance of proper training and regular practice.

Keeping Your Family Safe is essential reading for all who choose to use a gun for safety—and in safety.

Arthur Z. Berg, M.D.
Distinguished Life Fellow
American Psychiatric Association

Assistant Professor
Harvard Medical School
Massachusetts General Hospital

Acknowledgements

The authors thank Brian Kennedy, President of the Claremont Institute, for his support of the project Doctors for Responsible Gun Ownership. We are indebted to A.J. Cummings, MD for introducing us and making possible our collaboration as coauthors. Professor Dan Palm, Stephen P. Wenger, PharmD, and Teresa Wrobbel, MD lent their expertise in political philosophy, lead exposure control, and shooting during pregnancy. We have tried to reflect the knowledge we have acquired as students of Massad Ayoob, perhaps the most eloquent commentator on the verities of human aggression and a renowned teacher of self-defense.

John Holschen of InSights Training, LLC, Inc. in Bellingham, Washington contributed his skills in firearm handling and defensive techniques. John shares his experience as a U.S. Army Special Forces A-team operator and medic in training our civilian, military, and law enforcement personnel. Engineer and firearms expert John Gilman from Corvallis, Oregon, also contributed to our work.

Dr. Wipfler thanks his family, especially his parents, who taught him respect for others, a zest for life, and the duty of parents to protect their family. Growing up in a family and community where firearms are considered everyday tools for sport, recreation, and family self-defense has enabled Dr. Wipfler to appreciate the many benefits and significant responsibilities of firearm ownership.

Finally we thank our patient and indulgent wives RoseAnn Wheeler and Diane Wipfler for their support during our writing of this book. The best reward for our work that we can imagine is that it would prevent even one injury or death.

Chapter 1

The Facts About Firearms

Firearm ownership is deeply imbedded in America's history and traditions. From colonial times until the 1960s, keeping firearms for sport and self-defense was not controversial. The rifle over the fireplace, dad's hunting shotgun, and even the revolver in the bedside stand were familiar landmarks on the cultural landscape. Fathers and sons, even mothers and daughters of earlier times took their cue from America's founders, who wrote extensively about the role of firearms in national and family security.[1]

In an August 1785 letter to his nephew Peter Carr, Thomas Jefferson wrote, "A strong body makes the mind strong. As to the species of exercise, I advise the gun. While this gives a moderate exercise to the body, it gives boldness, enterprise, and independence to the mind."[2]

Over the years, as the population became more concentrated in cities, many Americans lost touch with the tradition of gun ownership. Some gradually assumed what they believed to be a progressive view that gun ownership is quaint and outdated, if not downright scary. Lurid media coverage of gun crimes reinforced a bad image of guns and gun owners, even though violent crimes in general have shown a long-term downward trend,[3] and fatal gun accidents are becoming rare.[4]

Although firearms played a vital part in America's founding and history, they have become controversial in some circles. Some medical practitioners have promoted a view, often colored by emotion, of firearms as inherently dangerous.[5] This view has become less accepted as a large body of scientific evidence has developed showing firearms to be very safe in responsible hands. In particular, it has become clear that children who are introduced to firearms by a trained family member live in a world apart from the stereotyped juvenile delinquent who only learns the misuse of guns from similarly misguided peers on the street.

A 1994 study published by the U.S. Department of Justice's Office of Juvenile Justice and Delinquency Prevention found that

> Boys who own legal firearms, however, have much lower rates of delinquency and drug use and are even slightly less delinquent than nonowners of guns. The socialization into gun ownership is also vastly different for legal and illegal gunowners. Those who own legal guns have fathers who own guns for sport and hunting. On the other hand, those who own illegal guns have friends who own illegal guns and are far more likely to be gang members. For legal gunowners, socialization appears to take place in the family; for illegal gunowners, it appears to take place "on the street."[6]

The discovery that a family's protective guidance teaches children to be safe with guns should surprise no one. That is what a family is for—to give a child the tools to negotiate life's challenges with confidence and responsibility. Generations of American families have brought up their children with respect for the duties and power that come with owning a gun.

Just as families teach their children well, so do communities. Countless local and state firearm associations across the United States hold regular youth shooting events for competitors aged 10 through 20 years. Junior rifle clubs thrive even in states whose governments are generally hostile to gun owners. For example, the Association of New Jersey Rifle & Pistol Clubs has 63 member clubs around the state. Two of these are gun clubs exclusively for juniors.[7]

This association's members volunteer their weekends and donate their money for New Jersey's young people. They award two $1,500 scholarships each year to high school seniors or new graduates. Its annual YouthFest offers kids and their parents a day at the range to try rifle and shotgun shooting under the watchful guidance of NRA-certified instructors. Newcomers quickly learn that the prejudices against guns and gun owners they may have learned from popular sources are unfair and unjustified.

The California Rifle and Pistol Association (CRPA) conducts four major youth shooting championships each year, each in a separate small-bore firearm competition.

National education programs reinforce and augment these state and local institutions. The National Rifle Association (NRA) devotes enormous resources to women's programs that include training in firearm safety, target shooting, hunting, and self-defense. The NRA's Youth Programs sponsor shooting events around the country, often in conjunction with local shooting clubs. Its annual Youth Education Summit in Washington, D.C. provides scholarships for exceptional high school students to spend a week studying the political process and the significance of the Constitution and Bill of Rights.

The National Shooting Sports Foundation (NSSF) has taken a leading role in teaching families about responsible firearm ownership. As the premier firearm industry group, the NSSF has a practical interest in seeing that firearms are used safely and responsibly. Toward that goal, the NSSF publishes online and print brochures on gun safety and hunting ethics and a parent's guide to recreational shooting for youngsters.[8]

Every part of this educational network—from parent to youth shooting club to national organization—has one vital feature in common. They all emphasize the absolute necessity of adult involvement in teaching kids about guns. Whether it's a father taking his daughter out to the range or an Olympic youth shooting team coach steering a gifted young marksman to victory, the adult imparts to his young students the foundation lessons of life.

Of course, the young shooters learn all the basics of gun safety, which we will cover in detail in this book. And they learn how to shoot well by learning how to hold the firearm, how to align the sights, and how to control the trigger. But they also learn self-discipline. They realize in vivid terms how destructive a firearm can be if handled carelessly, and how terribly immoral it is to hurt someone wrongfully with a gun.

Young students of the shooting sports learn how training—the rote and sometimes tedious repetition of simple tasks—can make them excel. They learn persistence, teamwork, and respect for their teachers and fellow shooters. These are all life lessons for growth and maturity, lessons they would never learn from their peers on the street.

Parents will recognize in this recitation of good habits the goals of many youth activities, including team sports, the study of music, and more. But the shooting sports provide a grounding in all the virtuous lessons we listed above, plus one unique benefit. They make the child immune to the dangerous lure of playing with guns. In a world where it is impossible to shield your child from all dangers, it makes sense to give him or her the tools to avoid them, or at least to manage them effectively. Just as we teach kids to swim, we can teach them the handling firearms in a gradual, trusting, and totally safe manner.

Every junior shooter studies and practices under the close supervision of trained adult instructors. Being emotionally settled is a prerequisite for consistent accuracy in shooting, because concentration is crucial. Youth trainers teach the notion of a Zen-like "inner position" that must be attained by the student who expects to shoot accurately.

The idea that mental discipline and maturity can be instilled in kids through organized shooting sports seems odd to those who only hear bad things about kids and guns. A steady media diet of juvenile crime stories and overblown portrayals of the few tragic fatal gun accidents seem to say that kids and guns never mix. But we know from hundreds of years' experience that not only can young people learn how to be safe with guns, they can learn how to be mature and responsible citizens by learning shooting skills.

The September 11, 2001 attacks on America abruptly reminded families of the need for national and personal security. Watching the twin towers of the World Trade Center fall in flames and seeing the Pentagon attacked dispelled the illusion of invulnerability for most of us. The good side of this tragedy is that America seems to have renewed the faith of our founders that we are responsible for our own defense, both as a nation and as individuals.

This book intends to answer questions that have arisen in the minds of Americans who are taking a fresh look at owning guns for personal and family security. How can I assure my family's safety from crime? Can I legally use a gun to defend my family? Can I own a gun under existing laws? Is it even morally right to own guns? We hope to give our readers a solid foundation of knowledge in all these areas. After reading this book, some may decide that gun ownership is not for them. We respect that decision, and only ask that they recognize the vital part it surely plays in the lives of many other American families.

But all who read this book will be provided with an opportunity to understand that firearm ownership is their heritage and their right. They will also know how to assert that right safely and responsibly in their homes and communities.

ENDNOTES

1. "How Did the Founders Understand the Second Amendment?" compiled by Palm, D. in Palm D, Wheeler T (ed), *A Citizen's Guide to the Second Amendment*, The Claremont Institute 2002.

2. *Letters, Thomas Jefferson 1743-1826*, University of Virginia Electronic Text Library, http://etext.lib.virginia.edu/etcbin/toccer-new2?id=JefLett. sgm&images=images/modeng&data=/texts/english/modeng/parsed&tag =public&part=32&division=div1 .

3. Stolinsky D, Wheeler T. *Firearms: A Handbook for Health Professionals*. The Claremont Institute, Claremont, California (1999): 11-12.

4. *Injury Facts—2001 Edition on CD-ROM*, National Safety Council, Itasca, Illinois 2001: 40-41.

5. Adelson L, "The Gun and the Sanctity of Human Life; or The Bullet as Pathogen", *Archives of Surgery* 127 (1992): 659-664.

6. "Urban Delinquency and Substance Abuse: Initial Findings," Office of Juvenile Justice and Delinquency Prevention, U.S. Department of Justice, Office of Justice Programs (March 1994), page 18. http://www.ncjrs.org/pdffiles/urdel.pdf.

7. Association of New Jersey Rifle & Pistol Clubs, *News & Briefs* 19, no. 4 (July/August 2007): 13.

8. National Shooting Sports Foundation web site, http://www.nssf.org. Family should be involved with planning and preparedness.

Chapter 2

How to Use this Book

As practicing physicians the authors have a natural inclination to emphasize safety. Keeping your family safe with guns in the home is a sensible goal of public health education, one we feel uniquely qualified to teach. Although other physicians and medical organizations have claimed to teach gun safety, their efforts have often been clouded by political attitudes hostile to gun ownership. Of even greater concern is the tendency of some medical organizations to urge doctors to tell families not to own guns at all, that they are too dangerous.

No doctor should ever misuse the trust of a patient to promote a political position against gun ownership. For a doctor to bring politics into the exam room is a form of unprofessional physician conduct known as an ethical boundary violation.[1] When the politics are intended to make patients get rid of their guns, the violation is even worse, since it is intended to erode the patient's constitutional right to own firearms.

Ethical considerations aside, for all the reasons detailed in the first chapter of this book, we know such advice to be wrong. Safety is achievable for those willing to seek the proper training and equipment. Technology has given us secure locking mechanisms that keep guns inaccessible to children and unauthorized adults yet allow rapid access within seconds if the need should drastically arise.

Every American who is law-abiding and levelheaded can handle firearms perfectly safely. And as good citizens of this great country, you have the right to own firearms. Only by deliberate or reckless abuse of that right can it legitimately be taken away from you.

Those who may not be familiar with firearms, and therefore may feel uneasy around them, are just as entitled to own them as the most enthusiastic target shooter. It is toward this group, newcomers with a desire to learn more, that we direct this book. The book itself provides all the basic information a family with no knowledge of guns needs to become competent and safe with firearms in their home. They will know the different kinds of firearms in use today, the basic workings of each, how to load, shoot, unload, clean, and safely store any firearm they choose to own.

Beginners will also be introduced to the ethics and law of self-defense. Much false information surrounds these topics, even though they are well grounded in a long tradition of American law. Any responsible gun owner is capable of learning and applying the law regarding self-defense, and in fact has a duty to learn it.

After learning some of the basic legal requirements of firearm ownership, the reader will learn where he or she can learn how to shoot. In addition to the local, state, and national resources for shooting instruction listed in the first chapter, we will provide information on further resources for firearm training. These resources can take the student of firearms as far as he could ever want to go—to Olympic competition, to advanced levels of tactical competence, or to a challenging and satisfying hobby for the whole family.

Others may have some familiarity with firearms, but would like a refresher in safety. They may already have firearms and use them for hunting or target shooting. Or they may own firearms for home defense, but would like to feel more secure in their abilities. The chapters on safety, training, and self-defense should be especially valuable to these intermediate shooters.

Some readers may already be expert in one or more shooting disciplines. This group would include the experienced hunter, the devoted target shooter, and even the graduate of shooting instruction courses. The range of shooting activities and skills is so diverse that no one masters them all. For this group of specialists we hope to offer a broad perspective they may not have encountered. In addition to the family benefits of gun ownership, these readers may encounter for the first time a discussion of the ethics and laws of self-defense.

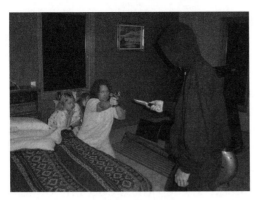

Although statistically a rare event, many break-and-entry criminal attacks have been stopped by armed citizens who have taken the time to get the right equipment, training, and maintain their skills.

In recent years the laws of many states have changed to allow citizens to take responsibility for their own safety from criminal assault. The people of these states have come to the realization that law-abiding, mentally competent citizens can be trusted to carry personal firearms for defense of family and self. Since 1987, when Florida became the first state to pass a law enabling widespread concealed carry, detailed crime statistics have proved concealed carry license holders to be exceedingly safe and law-abiding. In fact, the crime rate among license holders is consistently lower than that of the general population.

Accordingly, we will cover in detail the tactics and etiquette of carrying a concealed firearm for self-protection. Firearm tactics for self-defense in the home, in automobiles, and in the workplace will be useful to readers at all levels of expertise.

For all readers, from beginners to experts, we offer a list of resources for further learning. A section of suggested reading provides a world of knowledge about America's great tradition of firearm ownership and its political origins in England. A list of training schools will enable the adventurous to study shooting with the world experts. And the whole book will show the world of possibilities for every family to rediscover the uniquely American spirit of independence and self-reliance that made us what we are today.

Endnote

1. Wheeler T, "Boundary Violation: Gun Politics in the Doctor's Office", *Medical Sentinel 4*, no. 2 (March-April 1999): 60-61.

Chapter Three

Types of Firearms

What is a Firearm?

To understand our subject we should first address what we mean by firearms. Over history many weapons have been invented for the purpose of projecting an object for some distance. The spear, the bow and arrow, the catapult, and the musket are examples of the variety of such inventions. Today's military technology has given us an awe-inspiring range of weapons, from rocket-propelled grenades to intercontinental ballistic missiles with nuclear warheads. Special military weapons are designed for well-defined military objectives and are not suited for personal or home defense. They are not relevant to civilian firearm ownership, and so we will not discuss them further.

Merriam-Webster's 11th Collegiate Dictionary defines "firearm" as "a weapon from which a shot is discharged by gunpowder—usually used of small arms." The word dates back to 1646, and its definition still applies today. A firearm is not a bomb or a bazooka or a grenade launcher. It can be held and fired by one person, and it has the civilian uses of sport, hunting, and self-defense.

Air guns and guns powered by compressed gas have a place in some shooting sports, and the general rules of firearm safety apply to them as much as to firearms. However, they are not considered firearms and will not be relevant to our discussion.

All firearms for civilian use can be divided into three categories—rifles, shotguns, and handguns. Rifles and shotguns are sometimes collectively called long guns. Handguns in turn are divided into revolvers and pistols. Firearms all have a *stock* or *frame* that holds the parts together, an *action* that the shooter operates to load and fire a round, and a *barrel*, or metal tube designed for a particular size of cartridge. A small metal post or bead (the *front sight*) is built on the top of the barrel's muzzle end. To aim the gun, the shooter aligns it with a notch built on the top of the barrel's rear end (the *rear sight*). Instead of these "iron sights" a telescope, laser sight, or electronic projected-dot sight can be mounted on the barrel or frame for increased accuracy. Every firearm fires a projectile made of lead, or more recently for some guns steel, using the force created by controlled burning of gunpowder.

Some guns used by hobbyists still use the centuries-old technique of loading the powder charge and the bullet into the muzzle (the forward end) of the barrel. However, most modern rifles and handguns fire a *cartridge*, sometimes called a *round*. A cartridge is a self-contained little package consisting of four parts: the *case*, the *primer*, the *powder charge*, and the *bullet*. In shotguns the unit of ammunition is called a *shotgun shell* or *shotshell*. The case is a plastic shell with a metal base, or head. Most shotshells contain multiple lead or steel balls, called *shot*, although a single *slug* can be used as the projectile.

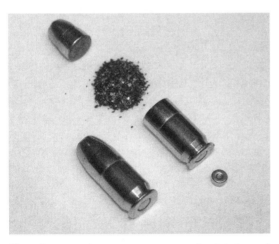

The four main components of pistol and rifle ammunition are the case, primer, gunpowder and bullet.

The case is a metal container adapted to fit into a particular gun. Tightly fitted into the base of the cartridge is a metal cup with a chemical that ignites the powder charge. A carefully measured amount of gunpowder, just right for the cartridge and gun, is contained in the case. Tightly fitted into the other end of the case is the bullet, the projectile that leaves the barrel of the gun when it's fired.

Each firing of a cartridge or round involves loading the round into the *chamber*, located in the *breech* of the barrel (or into the cylinder for revolvers). The breech is the end of the barrel closer to the shooter. Then the action is closed, securing the cartridge in the chamber, which is simply a reinforced, strong part of the breech exactly fitted to accept the cartridge. The closed chamber ensures that all the force of the firing will be directed down the barrel and out the *muzzle* (the end of the barrel where the bullet comes out).

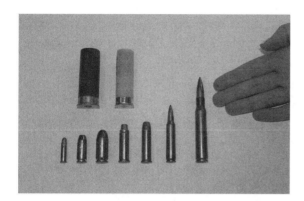

The following cartridges are included for size comparison and include from left to right the following: .22 long rifle rimfire, 9mm, .45 Auto, .38 Special, .357 Magnum, .223 (5.56mm), 30-06, and at the top are a 20-gauge shotgun (right) and 12-gauge shotgun shell (left).

When the cartridge has been loaded and the action closed, securing the cartridge in the chamber, the shooter then *cocks* the gun. This means the shooter draws the hammer or firing pin back, making it ready to be released by pulling the trigger. Most firearms other than revolvers are equipped with a *safety*. The safety is usually a small lever or slide located within the reach of the shooter's thumb or finger. It is placed in the "on" position to prevent firing of the gun when the shooter is not ready to fire, then moved to the "off" position when the shooter has placed the sights on the target and is ready to fire.

Most firearm actions combine the cocking action with the loading or firing action, so they occur with one step. But the Western style single action revolver, for example, requires the shooter to manually cock the gun for each shot by pulling back the hammer with the thumb.

When the shooter is ready and sure of the target, she pulls the trigger, releasing the hammer or firing pin, which is pushed forward by a spring into a small opening in the rear of the chamber and strikes the primer of the cartridge. The chemical in the primer then ignites, in turn igniting the powder. The powder then burns smoothly, producing a very rapidly expanding gas. It is the pressure of this expanding gas that pushes the bullet out of the case and down the barrel, out the muzzle and toward the target.

Once the bullet is fired, the empty cartridge with its spent primer is ejected. Depending on the type of gun this is done either manually by the shooter or automatically as part of the gun's firing sequence. The primer and bullet can be used only once, but most cartridge cases can be reloaded by inserting a new primer, powder charge, and bullet.

The .22 caliber round, popular for informal target shooting, is an exception. It has a non-reusable case. Its primer is applied to the inside surface of the case's rim, and not into a cup type of primer in the center of the base, or *case head*. Rifles and handguns chambered

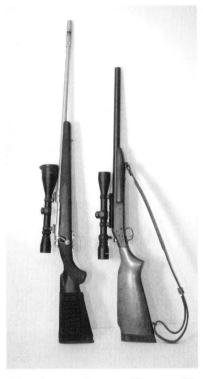

for the .22 caliber round have a firing pin designed to strike the rim of the case head, and not the center. Therefore it is called a *rimfire* cartridge, and the cartridge with a center-placed primer is a *centerfire* cartridge.

What is a Rifle?

A rifle is a long gun designed to shoot a single bullet in a single caliber, or diameter of bullet. Thus a .22 caliber rifle takes only (is chambered for) a .22 caliber cartridge, whose bullet measures .22 inch across. The rifle is inherently the most accurate firearm of the three types. It also is able to shoot accurately for longer distances than handguns or shotguns, that is, it has a longer range. Rifles come in a wide variety of calibers from the tiny, extremely accurate .17 caliber to the mighty .50 BMG caliber rifle.

Of these two rifles with telescopic sights, the one on the left is a bolt action rifle. The rifle on the right has a single shot break action.

Rifles are distinguished from shotguns by the presence of *rifling*, or spiral grooves machined into the barrel's inner surface. The ridges left between the grooves are called *lands*. A rifle's *bore* is the distance from one land to the land on the opposite side. Modern handguns also have rifled barrels. Rifling puts a spin on the bullet as it travels down the barrel. This spin stabilizes the course of the bullet, contributing to accuracy.

Rifles and shotguns also have several types of actions, or mechanisms for loading and firing the cartridge or shotshell.

The *bolt action* rifle uses a steel cylinder with a handle that is moved back and forth by the shooter for each shot. Opening the bolt extracts the spent cartridge case and cocks the action for the next shot. Closing the bolt carries a fresh live round forward and locks it securely in the chamber. The bolt action rifle is a good rifle for beginners because having to cycle the action manually for each shot teaches the shooter to make every shot count. The bolt type of action is also used in some shotguns.

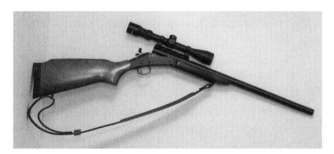

This single-shot break-action is opened and ready to load or unload. Note the sling attached which makes it easier to carry to carry over the shoulder.

The *pump* or *slide action* rifle uses a sliding portion of the forward end of the stock (the *forearm*) to do the work of ejecting the spent case, cocking the action, and chambering a new round. Between every shot the shooter moves the forearm to the rear and then back into its forward position. Shotguns also employ the slide action, as many hunting, police, and military shotguns demonstrate.

Hinge or *break actions* are used in shotguns and some rifles. Fine shotgun manufacturers are famous for their high-quality, expensive hunting shotguns that use the break action. This is perhaps the simplest type of action, requiring the shooter to break open the action to extract the spent shotshell by hand and load a new one. Many break action shotguns are double-barreled, with either a side-by-side or over-and-under barrel configuration.

The *lever action* uses a hand-operated lever on the underside of the rifle to open and close the action, to load rounds into the chamber and eject empty brass, and to cock the hammer. The lever action was used extensively in earlier rifle models and is characterized by the legendary Winchester Model 94 rifle, familiar to fans of Western movies and television shows. This style is still quite popular.

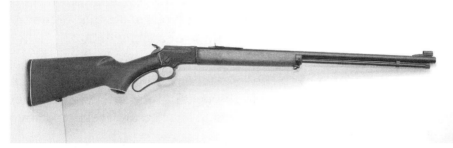

This lever action rifle was designed in the mid 1800s and remains a popular type of rifle.

A *semiautomatic* action uses energy from the cartridge firing to do the work of extracting, cocking, and loading. Ingenious engineering made possible the design of rifles, shotguns, and handguns with moving slides of various types. Whatever the specific design, every semiautomatic firearm harnesses part of the energy produced by the firing cartridge to push a sliding part to the rear, compressing a spring and recocking the action. Then the slide is driven forward by the spring, loading a new round into the chamber. The shooter has only to pull the trigger for each shot.

Modern police firearms almost all have semiautomatic actions. The advantages for these applications are rapid-fire capability and firepower, or the ability to fire multiple rounds without manually reloading. Semiautomatic firearms, like some bolt action and slide action firearms, all have a means of storing multiple rounds for rapid feeding into the chamber. For most semiautomatics this mechanism is the *magazine*, a detachable metal or polymer container into which cartridges are placed before a shooting session. Most rifle magazines fit into an opening or *magazine well* in front of the trigger assembly. For handguns, the magazine usually fits into the grip.

The empty or nearly empty magazine can be ejected and replaced with a fresh magazine in a few seconds, allowing nearly uninterrupted engagement of a target or multiple targets.

For completeness we mention firearms with an *automatic action*. These are the guns widely referred to as machine guns. They are very strictly regulated by federal law, and most automatic firearms owned by private citizens are used for target shooting and as collector's items.

The web site GunCite.com gives a useful summary of facts about machine guns (www.guncite.com/gun_control_gcfullau.html). A private citizen who wants to own a machine gun must apply to the federal government's Bureau of Alcohol, Tobacco, Firearms, and Explosives (BATFE), undergo a criminal background investigation by the FBI, and submit fingerprints and a photograph, and more. Some states forbid ownership of machine guns regardless of the federal law.

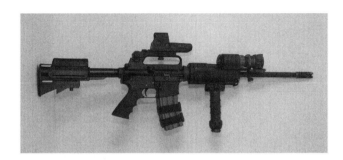

This semi-automatic rifle allows the shooter to fire a shot each time the trigger is pulled. This style is mistakenly maligned by some media sources without any factual basis.

Since 1934, only two legally owned machine guns have ever been used in a crime. In 1988, GunCite.com tells us, a Dayton, Ohio police officer used his legally owned machine gun to kill a police informant. The officer pleaded guilty to the crime and was sentenced to 18 years in prison. In the second case, also in Ohio, a doctor pleaded guilty and was sentenced to prison for the 1992 murder of another doctor with a machine gun.

Of course, some people with criminal intent acquire machine guns in spite of the strict federal and state laws. They don't feel obligated to submit to background checks, fingerprinting, being photographed, and all the other burdensome and intrusive measures that law-abiding people accept in becoming lawful machine gun owners. But even so, machine gun-toting criminals are relatively rare. Very few crime guns recovered by police are fully automatic weapons.

Practically all automatic firearms are rifles. They are used almost exclusively for military applications and as special police tactical

weapons. They have essentially no place in a comprehensive personal or home security plan.

An automatic action allows the bolt of the rifle to cycle repeat-
edly and very rapidly as long as the trigger is held down, or until
the magazine is emptied of ammunition. The Colt M4 rifle is the lat-
est version of the U.S. armed forces' light infantry rifle. It achieves
a cyclic rate of fire of 700 to 950 rounds per minute.[1] This highly
adaptable military weapon is equipped with a switch that allows
semiautomatic firing or fully automatic firing. The Colt M4 is a good
example of a selective-fire automatic rifle—technically known as an
assault rifle.

What is an "Assault Weapon"?

How does an assault rifle differ from an "assault weapon"? We
approach this question with no desire to enter the political conflict
that has raged for more than a decade about so-called assault weapons. However, we believe we owe our readers an accounting of the

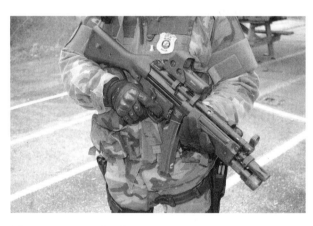

facts. There is no
such category of
firearms as assault
weapons. The term
"assault weapon"
was invented not
by military weapons
experts, but by jour-
nalists to describe
guns with a scary,
military appearance.
Outside this lim-
ited and politically
motivated sense,
the term "assault
weapon" is mean-
ingless. It is worse

This weapon is fully automatic, an HK MP-5
submachine gun. This one is used by a
Midwestern city tactical law officer in support of
the SWAT team.

than meaningless, because it accomplishes what its users intend—
to confuse and frighten the public into believing that these firearms
should be banned. For at least a hundred years military firearms,
including assault rifles, have been copied for use by civilians for target practice and collecting. The civilian version of the M4 military

rifle is the Match Target M4. To make this civilian version conform to federal laws restricting ownership of full-auto rifles, the selective fire feature of the M4 has been replaced with an action that only allows semiautomatic fire. It is this kind of gun, military in look but like any other target rifle in reality, that the journalists call assault weapons.

The profound confusion about what constitutes an assault weapon has been used to promote and pass legislation to label certain guns as assault weapons for the purpose of banning them. Criminalizing gun ownership according to the imagined threatening appearance of some firearms has had predictably bad results. For example, California law defines one characteristic of assault weapons as having a magazine that fits into the gun outside of the grip. Some fancy Olympic target pistols are designed this way—like the Walther pistols used by San Diego's Olympic-class teen shooting team, the Black Mountain

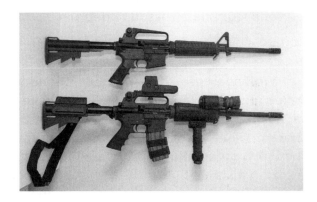

The M4 rifles seen here are present in factory issue (top) and sporterized with flashlight, EOTech sight, special sling and other special features. (bottom)

Shooting Club. Until red-faced California legislators quietly passed a law exempting the team, California's assault weapon law condemned these world-class junior shooters as "minors with assault weapons." Their coach could have gone to prison on a felony charge.

Without belaboring this unhappy situation any further, let us state a few facts about the guns maligned as assault weapons:

- Fewer than 2% of crime guns are so-called assault weapons.[2] Criminals prefer good quality handguns.

- The guns called assault weapons are no more dangerous than other firearms. Many common target and hunting rifles are far more powerful than "assault weapons."

• Many common firearms in production for years, seen frequently at target ranges and kept in the homes of many honest citizens, have been labeled assault weapons. Gun owners have been turned into status criminals because they unknowingly possess a gun that has arbitrarily been classified as an assault weapon.

We hope that by education the public will eventually understand that there are no bad guns. We assume that our readers are decent citizens who would never misuse a gun to harm an innocent human being. Yes, there are people who misuse guns, but that sad fact is never a legitimate reason to deprive the law-abiding of their rights.

What is a Shotgun?

We have seen that shotguns share many design features with rifles. Both are long guns, and they have nearly the same variety of action types. But shotguns differ from rifles mainly in the size of the bore, or diameter of the barrel, and the type of projectile they fire. The bore of a shotgun is considerably larger than that of a rifle. Instead of firing a single bullet, the shotgun typically fires with each round a group of small lead or steel balls, or shot. The shotgun can also fire a single large projectile called a shotgun slug or sabot. These are used in many states for hunting deer. This ability to handle a variety of ammunition makes the shotgun a versatile tool with a wide range of applications in hunting, target shooting, police work, and the military.

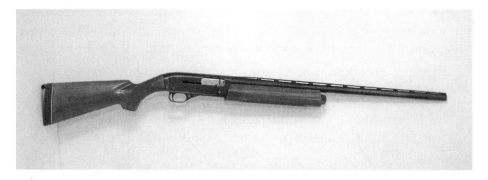

This semi-automatic 12 gauge shotgun is commonly used by hunters and sportsmen and also works very effectively when used for home defense. It holds 4 rounds in the tubular magazine plus one in the chamber.

Shotgun barrels do not have rifling and are said to be *smoothbore* barrels.

Shotgun bores are measured not in hundredths of an inch or in millimeters, as are rifle and handgun bores. The bore of a shotgun is measured by gauge. *Gauge* is calculated by the number of pure lead balls the exact size of the bore that it would take to weigh one pound. Modern shotguns come in 10-, 12-, 16-, 20-, and .410 gauge. The .410 gauge actually is a caliber designation, the only exception to the gauge measuring system.[3]

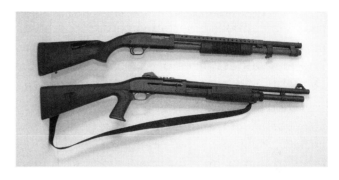

The bore of a shotgun barrel can be made with a constriction, or choke, toward the muzzle. These shotguns have pump or slide actions. The shotgun on the bottom has a pistol-grip style stock and sling that offers several advantages in tactical situations. Both hold a total of 9 rounds and are formidable home defense weapons.

The *choke* shapes the grouping of shot as the shot leaves the barrel and travels toward the target. A *cylinder choke* (also called an *open choke*) is actually no choke at all. The bore is the same diameter from breech to muzzle. Since the cylinder choke does not constrict the shot load at all, the shot scatters more than with any other choke.

The *improved cylinder choke* mildly constricts the shot group just before it leaves the barrel, producing a tighter (closer together) pattern of holes in the target. A *modified choke* constricts the shot group even further, producing an even tighter target pattern. The *full choke* keeps the shot group tightly together as it leaves the barrel, producing the tightest target pattern. Some shotguns can be fitted with an *adjustable choke*.

Another reason that shotguns are so versatile is the variety of sizes that shot comes in. Shot size is measured in hundredths of an inch, and each size is referred to by a number. Following the archaic and somewhat confusing system of shotgun terminology, the larger the number, the smaller the shot. The smallest shot is No. 9, measuring .08 inches in diameter. The next size larger is No. 8 ½, measuring

.085 inches. Then come Nos. 8, 7½, 6, 5, 4, 2, 1, BB, T, and F, which measures .22 inches.

A separate category of larger shot is called *buckshot*, which uses still a different numbering system. The smallest buckshot size is No. 4, which measures .24 inch in diameter. In order of increasing size the designations are No. 4, No. 3, No. 2, No. 1, 0, 00 (double aught), and 000 (triple aught) buckshot. No. 4 buckshot is slightly larger than .22 caliber. Imagine shooting 21 lead or steel balls in a single shot, each one a little bigger in diameter than a .22 caliber bullet. The four largest sizes of buckshot are comparable to rifle or pistol calibers. The largest size, No. 000, measures .36 caliber, or 0.36 inch diameter. There are 9 pellets of this size in a single shotshell.

Because of the great variety of gauges, chokes, and shot size, we cannot cover the whole range of shotgun uses in this book. More training is available for those readers who want to know more. We devote a separate chapter to firearm training in which local and national-level firearm education resources are discussed in detail.

What is a Handgun?

The third category of firearms is the *handgun*. A common name for all handguns is *pistol*, but this term has come to mean all handguns but *revolvers*. Handguns have come in many designs over the centuries, but today almost all handguns fall into two categories—the revolver and the semiautomatic.

The older design, still very popular, is the revolver. Revolvers have a frame, a barrel, a *cylinder*, and an action. The barrel screws into the frame and is for practical purposes part of the frame. The cylinder is a strong wheel-like rotating part that both holds cartridges (usually six) and serves as the chamber. To load a revolver, the shooter uses the thumb-operated *cylinder latch* on the side of the frame to unlock the cylinder and swing it out of the frame. The shooter then ejects any spent cartridge cases with a sharp push on the cylinder's *ejector rod*, and then inserts a fresh round into each chamber of the cylinder. Then the shooter swings the cylinder back up into place, locking it into the frame.

When the revolver is loaded and the cylinder is locked into the frame with the chamber aligned with the barrel, the revolver is ready to fire. Pulling the trigger turns the cylinder to align the next chamber (with a fresh live round) with the barrel, cocks the *hammer*, and then releases the hammer. The hammer's firing pin then strikes the primer, firing the round in the same way that a rifle or shotgun fires.

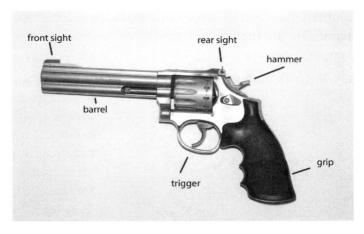

The revolver has several key parts that the owners should become familiar with in order to use it effectively for self defense..

This kind of revolver action is referred to as *double action* because pulling the trigger both cocks the hammer and releases it.

A *single action* revolver's trigger does not cock the hammer; it only releases the hammer after the shooter has manually cocked it. Single action revolvers were in common use during America's western expansion, and they still carry the aura of the Old West. A popular shooting sport is Cowboy Action Shooting, in which competitors dress as characters from the Old West—town marshals, schoolmarms, and desperadoes—and compete in target shooting. Single action revolvers are the handguns of choice for these fun filled and family-oriented competitions.

The semiautomatic handgun, or pistol, has become highly developed in the last 20 years. Innovations in polymer and metal technology have allowed lighter, more durable, and more dependable handguns to be

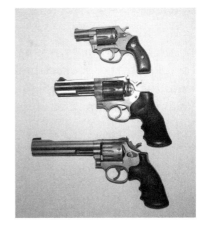

Revolvers some in a variety of sizes and styles. The barrel lengths of these double-action revolvers are 2, 4 and 6 inches. The firearm owner should consider their needs and personal preferences before purchasing a gun.

manufactured than ever before. Competition from overseas manufacturers has prompted the development of a dazzling variety of semiautomatics.

But all semiautomatics have the same basic components—a frame,

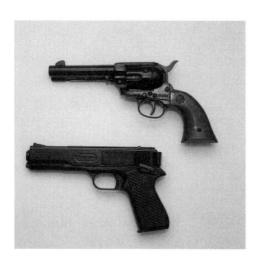

a barrel, a *slide*, an action, and a magazine. The frame houses the action, which uses either an exposed hammer or an enclosed firing pin to strike the cartridge primer. The magazine is detachable and fits into the magazine well in the butt or grip of the pistol.

Semiautomatic handguns designed throughout most of the 20th century could be classified as either single action or double action. These action types are quite different from the revolver actions of the same names. The single action semiauto-

The upper gun is a single-action revolver and the lower gun is a semiautomatic pistol.

matic requires only a very light and short trigger pull, just enough to release the cocked hammer. The double action semiautomatic requires a heavier and longer trigger pull, first to cock the action and second to release the hammer or firing pin.

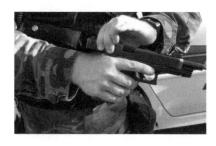

Instead of the semiautomatic rifle's bolt that travels back and forth, the semiautomatic handgun has a slide. The slide is a moving metal cover over the barrel, mounted on rails on the sides of the frame. The slide on some pistols is mounted inside the frame. When the trigger is pulled, energy from the fired cartridge forces the slide to the rear, ejecting the spent cartridge case and cocking the firing

The semi-automatic pistol here has the slide pulled back allowing confirmation that the gun is either loaded or unloaded.

pin or hammer. Then the slide, pushed by a spring, moves forward, stripping a fresh round off the stack of cartridges in the magazine, pushing it forward into the chamber, and locking the chamber again.

Each type of action has its advantages and disadvantages. The lighter and shorter trigger pull of the single action semiautomatic

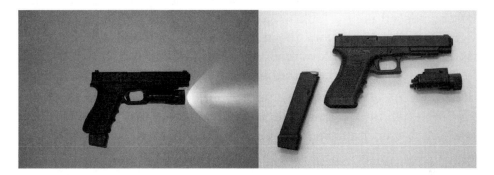

The handguns above are semiautomatic Glock pistols. The picture on the right shows the firearm with the 17 round magazine and flashlight detached. The picture on the left shows the gun with the light on. Many self-defense situations occur in darkness, and a flashlight is essential to proper threat identification and to assist with accurate shot placement.

makes it easier to shoot accurately. It allows faster repeat shots. But it requires more training and expertise to carry and shoot safely. For this reason law enforcement agencies mostly prefer pistols with the heavier and longer trigger pull of double action semiautomatics. The Glock pistol takes this evolution a step further, incorporating a safety lever into the trigger itself. Pulling the Glock trigger disengages the safety, completes the process of cocking the action, and releases the firing pin. This unique design, neither single nor double action, is called Safe Action by the manufacturer.

Military special forces units and some police special weapons and tactics (SWAT) teams prefer the single action pistol's accuracy and rapid-fire capability. The extra training required to use these pistols properly fits with the intensive training protocols of these specialized units.

Like rifles and shotguns, handguns come in a wide variety of calibers. They range from the .17 HMR cartridge through the mid-range 9 millimeter and .40 Smith & Wesson to the massive .500 S & W Magnum. Beginning handgun shooters do best with the .22

caliber handgun. This small round offers almost no recoil and allows the shooter to concentrate better on stance, grip, sight picture, sight alignment, and trigger control—the elements of accuracy. Once these basic elements are mastered, it is easier to adapt them to more powerful handguns.

This overview of the workings and terminology of firearms should be considered only a foundation. It is presented in general terms, with no effort to explore the many varied details of every firearm type. But it should allow readers to begin firearm training with an understanding of the basic equipment and how it works.

Before proceeding to training though, every gun owner must learn the habits that make shooting injury-free. We devote the next chapter to this vital lesson.

Endnotes

1. Colt's Manufacturing Co. web site, http://www.colt.com/mil/M4_2.asp.

2. Kleck G. *Targeting Guns: Firearms and Their Control*, Aldine de Gruyter, New York 1997: 112, 141.

3. California Hunter Education Manual, California Department of Fish and Game, Outdoor Empire Publishing, Inc., Seattle, Washington 1987: 23.

Chapter Four

Firearm Safety

For people unfamiliar with firearms, fear is the main obstacle to owning one. They understandably worry that somehow a terrible injury or even death could happen just because a gun is kept in the house. A constant barrage of news stories about gun accidents makes this concern seem real. But looking at the actual figures on firearm accidents should greatly relieve anyone who is looking into becoming a firearm owner. It is a fact that fatal firearm injuries have been slowly decreasing for over 70 years. This decrease in number (not just percentage) has occurred even as the population has more than doubled[1] and the number of guns owned by civilians has increased by five times.[2]

This unfamiliarity with firearms greatly enhances the perception of their risk. We tend to fear more those risks we don't know well. For example, more Americans die each year in swimming pool drownings than die from gun accidents, even though guns are far more numerous than swimming pools.[3] Yet we think of a swimming pool as a valued recreational feature of a happy home, even as we accept the risk of death it carries.

There is no shortage of dependable knowledge about gun accidents. Criminologists, the social scientists who study crime and criminal misuse of firearms, also study what kinds of people and situations are associated with firearm accidents. They find consistently that gun accidents, like other kinds of accidents, mostly happen to people with a pattern of habitual reckless behavior. These people often have poor driving records and records of arrests for offenses involving violence and alcohol abuse.[4] They represent the exact opposite of the attitudes and values that we will present in this chapter.

We will discuss the basic rules of firearm safety that apply to all applications of firearms. Whether a gun owner is a weekend target shooter, an Olympic-class rifle marksman, a police officer, or just a regular citizen, following these simple rules will all but eliminate the chance of a gun being fired accidentally.

As we progress through this chapter, think about the news reports of gun accidents you have read or heard recently. These stories invariably report that a gun was left lying out unsecured, so a child could pick it up. Or someone was pointing an "unloaded" gun at a friend or family member in play, only to find out the gun was loaded after all. Each accident was completely preventable, and in each case, one or more of the five rules of firearms handling was broken.

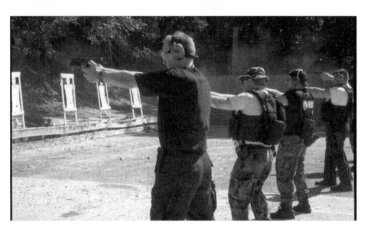

Part of becoming a responsible gun owner is learning to trust yourself with firearms. This self-confidence and feeling of proficiency is one of the satisfying benefits of learning gun safety. When you have learned the five basic rules, the reckless scenarios we described above will be unthinkable for you. You will know by reflex how to handle a gun safely.

Proficiency with firearms will come only after multiple trips to the shooting range.

The more advanced student of gun safety will also find special rules that apply to limited circumstances. For example, firing ranges and gun clubs generally have a list of house rules specific to that facility. A typical range rule is to stay behind a line painted along the firing line during the cease-fire. Some ranges allow the carrying of loaded handguns, but they must be holstered at all times unless one is actually shooting. Others require that any firearms not being fired be unloaded. There are good reasons for all these rules in their particular settings.

In this book we will keep to the basic rules that all must follow to be safe with firearms. There are only five rules, and we shall cover each one in detail.

The Five Rules of Gun Safety

Rule One—Treat every firearm as if it were loaded.

This rule is a mindset, a way of thinking seriously about guns. Following this rule means choosing the proper frame of mind for avoiding an accidental discharge, or unintentional firing of a round. Some firearm instructors teach that every accidental discharge is the result of negligence, and they prefer the term negligent discharge. But this term dismisses any possibility of equipment malfunction, which although rare, can occur. It is wrong to automatically condemn as negligent a shooter who has an accidental discharge if the cause lies in a faulty firearm. Improperly using the label of "negligent discharge" may also help a plaintiff's attorney establish negligence where none really occurred. Negligence is a key legal concept in deciding against a defendant in an accidental shooting. For these reasons we prefer the term accidental discharge.

By definition, firearm accidents occur without malice and without the shooter intending to harm anyone. The accidental discharge is unexpected. The shooter also often violates other rules, such as pointing the gun at someone while playing. A casual attitude toward handling firearms is a setup for tragedy. Faithfully following Rule One is the same as respecting the power of a firearm and resolving to use it properly at all times. Clearly, if you consider every firearm to be loaded you will never treat it as if it were unloaded and therefore safe to be careless with.

Rule Two—Never point a firearm at anything you are not willing to destroy.

This is strong language. It is intended to convey the truth that your gun could do great damage if you discharge it while it is pointed at the wrong thing. The damage could be as relatively trivial as punching a hole in the door of your hunting truck (although that would be bad enough), or as horrible as injuring or even killing a human being.

But if you can cause great and lasting damage by violating this rule, the opposite is just as true. It is quite comforting to realize that if you don't point the firearm at a particular object, you most certainly will never shoot it.

This rule applies even to a fraction of a second when the muzzle may be covering a person. For example, you may "sweep" a fellow shooter with your muzzle as you bring your gun around to aim at a target. It is helpful to think of a laser beam coming out of the muzzle of your gun. If your imaginary laser beam would hit anything you do not wish to shoot, even for a split second, then you are violating Rule Two. Following this rule is also called muzzle control.

Rule Three—Keep your finger off the trigger until your sights are on the target and you have made the decision to shoot.

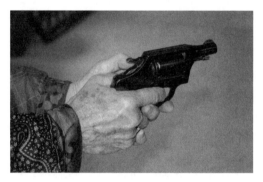

In this photograph, the gun owner has either wrongly placed her finger on the trigger or has consciously decided to shoot the gun and is in the process of squeezing the trigger. DO NOT PLACE YOUR FINGER ON THE TRIGGER UNTIL IT IS TIME TO SHOOT!

This is the most frequently violated rule. As a new shooter picks up a gun, he tends naturally enough to put his index finger on the trigger. It may seem awkward at first to hold a gun without resting the finger on the trigger. But long experience has shown that accidental discharges result most commonly from violations of Rule Three.

Even experienced police officers have violated Rule Three, often when stressed by a life-threatening encounter with a suspect. The stress of such a situation, whether for a police officer apprehending a dangerous criminal or a homeowner defending his family, can easily result in an unintentional discharge if the shooter's finger is on the trigger at the wrong time. The startle reflex causes muscles to suddenly contract, resulting in the fingers being instinctively flexed or tightened. If the finger is already positioned on the trigger, a loud noise or other startling event may cause an unintentional discharge of the gun with unwanted consequences.

Part of police and civilian tactical training is the repetitive and studied move of drawing and gripping a firearm while keeping the trigger finger outside the trigger guard. Generally this means the index finger is held straight along the frame of the gun.

If popular media are any indication, Rule Three is seeing more widespread adoption. News photos and movie portrayals of soldiers and police carrying service firearms increasingly show the trigger finger extended along the frame, in the safe position.

InSights Training, Inc. instructor and expert marksman John Holschen teaches that you should place your finger on the trigger only after you have made a conscious decision to fire the weapon. After that decision is made, the finger can be moved to the trigger in a fraction of a second.

After enough experience in handling firearms you will acquire a "muscle memory" for the right moves. It will become automatic when you pick up a gun to put your finger along the frame instead of inside the trigger guard. To put your finger on the trigger before you are ready to shoot will feel dangerously unnatural.

It is possible for some guns to discharge without the trigger being pulled. Older handgun designs sometimes resulted in accidental discharges when the gun had a round in the chamber and was dropped on its muzzle. The inertia of forward motion caused the firing pin to continue forward as the rest of the gun (and cartridge) stopped, causing the round to discharge. Newer designs have eliminated the problem of accidental firing when the handgun is dropped, but many of the older designs are still around and in good working order. It is always wise to be familiar with the particular make and model of any gun you use. Reading the manufacturers' manual may be optional for setting up your home entertainment center, but it is mandatory for learning how to operate your firearm safely.

Following Rule Three will make it virtually impossible to shoot anything but your intended target. If your sights are on your target and you are ready to shoot, then putting your finger on the trigger only at that time will prevent shooting at the wrong time.

Rule Four—Always be sure of your target and what is beyond it.

A bullet, once it leaves the barrel, cannot be recalled. If you have diligently followed the first three rules and properly fired your gun, then your bullet will hit what you fired at. But is it the right target? Are you sure that looming figure in the half-dark was an intruder with a gun, or is it a family member returning at an unexpected time or location? You must properly identify the person and the threat must be evident before you pull the trigger. To shoot before you are sure of a lethal threat can result in a nightmare.

This rule is also vitally important for the hunter, who shoots at targets in variable and often less than perfect weather and lighting conditions. Firing a round before a game target is positively identified can result in shooting livestock, hunting dogs, and worse. Just as important is to know where your bullet will come to rest if it does not stop in the target, or if you miss. Overpenetration of fired rounds is an ever-present challenge for law enforcement agencies. Much research has gone into designing defensive ammunition powerful enough to stop a lethal threat, but not so powerful that it exits the target and goes on to do unintended damage to persons or property. Law enforcement agencies must always guard

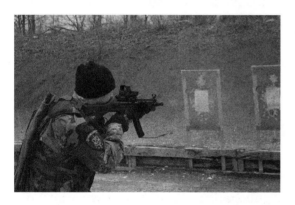

A quality firing range with a good backstop allows safe firearms practice. Rule 4 is to always be certain of your target and what is beyond it.

against the tendency of fired rounds to over-penetrate and strike unintended persons after the bullet passes through the criminal.

Several years ago, a SWAT unit in a large city surrounded a suspect, who began shooting. The order was given for the marksman with a high-powered rifle to shoot, and he hit his intended target. Unfortunately, the entry team of fellow SWAT officers had crept around to the other side of the small house. One of them was killed by the single bullet after it passed through the suspect, through the two walls of the house and out the other side, where it struck the officer.

Civilians should also be aware of the risk of over-penetration. A family living in a duplex or apartment may wish to choose a defensive firearm than has less penetration through drywall or other common building materials. Similarly, powerful hunting cartridges can cause great damage if a hunter does not ensure that a bullet will stop either in the intended target or in a safe backstop, such as a bank or hillside.

A properly designed shooting range makes it easy to follow Rule Four. The direction of fire always is toward a safe backstop, and the targets are clearly set up and identified before the shooter is allowed to fire or even pick up the firearm.

Rule Five—Always maintain complete control of your firearm.

You have a moral and legal obligation to control where your firearm is and who has access to it. This rule applies every minute of every day. It applies whether your gun is in your home, at your workplace, such as a small business with late hours, or on your person.

This rule is fairly new. It comes from an increasing understanding of how unintentional shootings occur and its gradual incorporation into state laws and court decisions. At least one reason for the marked decline in fatal gun accidents over the years is the teaching and implementation of basic gun safety. Some credit is undoubtedly due to an increased awareness among gun owners of the importance of preventing access of small children and other unqualified persons to firearms. Several states have passed laws defining negligent firearm storage. These laws, often referred to as *CAP (child access prevention) laws*, provide severe penalties for gun owners if they fail to store their guns properly and someone is wrongfully shot as a result.

We strongly recommend that any gun owner or prospective gun owner become familiar with the laws governing proper transportation and storage of firearms. These laws vary widely from one state to another. In some states it is quite easy to violate a law unknowingly by storing your gun in the wrong type of container when you travel. In Chapter 6 we will describe some proven techniques of proper firearm storage. These methods help the gun owner always to maintain complete control of his or her firearm.

Eye and Ear Protection

Firearms are some of the safest consumer items in common use. Firearm sports, as we have discussed, are some of the most injury-free. But these good records of safety depend on a culture of safety among responsible gun owners. In addition to the rules designed to prevent accidental shootings, we have safety rules for preventing non-shooting injuries.

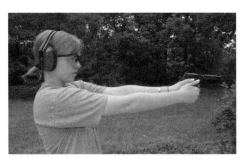

The new shooter is properly using eye and ear protection during firearms practice.

Foremost among these non-shooting injuries are damage to a shooter's hearing and penetrating injuries to the eyes. Fortunately eye injuries are uncommon, and proper eye protection makes them rare. Hearing damage is far more common. Greater awareness of the hearing damage caused by industrial and recreational noise has made hearing protection a standard safety rule at shooting ranges.

Metal plate targets commonly used in some pistol competitions can cause *ricochet*, or bouncing of a bullet or bullet fragments. Shooting clay targets can result in small clay fragments blowing or ricocheting toward the shooter. Semiautomatic firearms sometimes eject spent cases in the general direction of the shooter or toward a fellow shooter. Rarely, a defective round of ammunition can rupture, or a damaged firearm can allow escape of gases or metal fragments at high speed.

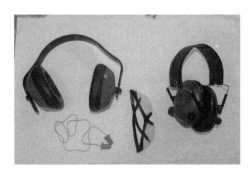

There are several styles of hearing and eye protection and they are essential to safe firearms use.

Some revolvers eject gas and particles of gunpowder backwards, causing a hazard to the shooter's eyes. On a typical target range firing line other shooters are positioned immediately to one's right or left side. Flying cartridge cases, lead shavings, and gunpowder particles from their guns can be as much of a danger to your eyes as the one from your own gun.

Cleaning your gun after shooting often requires some disassembly, or *field stripping*, of the gun (always follow the directions in the owner's manual). The springs found in semiautomatic firearms can slip loose and cause eye injury if not carefully controlled during field stripping. Droplets of cleaning fluid can cause eye irritation. Wearing eye protection is therefore mandatory while cleaning your gun.

Properly designed protective eyewear almost completely eliminates the possibility of eye injuries from these sources. The most common lens material is the tough plastic polycarbonate. The best lens design is the wrap-around type that provides protection from projectiles coming from the side as well as the front. Many eye protection products are available through sporting goods stores and firearms dealers.

Even the small .22 caliber cartridge discharges with enough noise to damage hearing. The medium and large calibers, not to mention shotguns, all cause a very loud and sudden noise that the human ear is not able to process without damage.

We measure the loudness of sound by the pressure of sound waves. Sound waves are a form of energy transmitted through the air. The sound energy sets the eardrum into motion, and a chain of delicate bones connects the eardrum to the even more delicate organ of hearing in the inner ear.

We measure sound energy (perceived as loudness) in *decibels*, abbreviated as dB. Here is a table of common sounds with their sound energy levels[5]:

Approximate Decibel	Example Level
0 dB	Faintest sound heard by human ear
30 dB	Whisper, quiet library
60 dB	Normal conversation, sewing machine, typewriter
90 dB	Lawn mower, shop tools, truck traffic
100 dB	Chain saw, pneumatic drill, snowmobile
115 dB	Sandblasting, loud rock concert, auto horn
140 dB	Gun muzzle blast, jet engine; noise causes pain

Hearing damage can occur from sound levels over 85 decibels if the exposure is repeated or sustained, for example, working around shop tools every day for 8 hours. But exposure of the unprotected ear to the noise of even one high-power rifle shot can cause permanent and irreparable hearing loss.

Hearing protection cannot completely block out the loud impact noise of a gunshot, but it can reduce the energy to a level much less likely to cause damage to hearing. The noise-blocking ability of ear protection products is called the *noise reduction rating*. This rating is the number of decibels by which the product reduces the noise heard by the protected ear.

The two types of hearing protectors are earplugs and earmuffs. Both types offer noise reduction ratings of about 15 to 30 dB. Wearing both plugs and muffs gives 10 to 15dB more protection than either type worn alone. The American Academy of Otolaryngology-Head and Neck Surgery advises wearing both plugs and muffs for protection against sound levels over 105 dB.[6] This would include the noise made by any caliber of firearm, even the little .22 caliber.

Plugs should be of the foam type, not the waxy type used to keep water out of the ears. The foam earplug is a little cylinder or blunt-pointed plug that the wearer first compresses between the finger and thumb, rolling it into a thin shape that is quickly inserted into the ear canal. The foam then expands, conforming to the ear canal and sealing it. It is important to get a good seal by inserting the compressed plug into the ear canal before it expands. Inserting these plugs properly can be a little tricky, and improperly placed foam earplugs cannot protect the ear. A few people with very small or irregularly shaped ear canals may be unable to wear plugs and should use muffs instead. But properly inserted foam earplugs are an inexpensive way to achieve noise reduction ratings as high as 33 dB.

Earmuffs should fit snugly, with the pillows encircling both ears. Eyeglasses can interfere with the proper fit of the muffs and impair their effectiveness. Because of the inherent limitations of both muffs and plugs, it is especially advisable to wear both types together when shooting.

In recent years a new type of hearing protection has become available. Electronic components in the muffs or plugs allow the wearer to hear sounds like conversation, range commands, and game animals, but to block the impact noise of gunfire. These products are especially useful in special situations like hunting, where safety requires being able to hear environmental sounds. Prices for these sophisticated products can run into several hundred dollars.

The risk of eye and hearing damage can never be completely eliminated, any more than the risk of injury from driving. For regular shooters, a hearing test done every year or two by an audiologist is a good idea, since hearing protection is not perfect. But a habit of wearing good quality protection should give shooters confidence that their eyes and ears are safe.

Lead Exposure

Lead is the traditional metal for making bullets. It is malleable, heavy, and easily melted, all qualities that make it suitable for ammunition. However, it is also chemically similar to elements the body incorporates into tissues and uses in essential biochemical functions. That makes it potentially poisonous. But lead poisoning generally requires repeated and prolonged exposure to a significant level of lead. Sensible precautions can protect shooters.

Shooters are exposed to lead particles from fired bullets. These are shavings coming off the bullet as it is fired, or as it hits a metal target. Another source of lead is the lead styphnate found in bullet primers. Protective measures prevent lead entry into the body by inhaling or swallowing lead residue.

Firearm trainer Stephen Wenger, who has a doctoral degree in pharmacy, advises several measures for reducing lead exposure. At indoor shooting ranges, wear a respirator or mask with a HEPA filter for lead. Properly designed indoor ranges have good ventilation, but even the best are more likely to expose a shooter to lead than an outdoor range. After shooting, wash your hands and face, including any facial hair, with soap and cool water. Do this before you leave the range if possible. Eating with lead residue on your face or hands obviously can increase the chance of swallowing the residue.

Wear a cap when shooting. Not only does this keep lead mist out of your hair, the bill keeps the occasional ejected cartridge case from getting caught between your eyeglasses and your face. The freshly ejected cartridge case is hot and can cause immediate pain and burns. The distraction can cause a shooter unintentionally to discharge an uncontrolled gun, resulting in injury to himself or others.

When you get home, change clothes as soon as convenient to prevent lead and soot from contaminating your home. When cleaning your guns, wear old clothes dedicated to that task or do this chore before changing from your shooting clothes. Cleaning the gun dislodges lead particles. You can also be possibly exposed to hazardous chemicals in your gun cleaning fluid, so clean your guns outdoors if possible. In any case, make sure the area is well ventilated. Wearing vinyl examination gloves further minimizes exposure to lead and cleaning chemicals.

Shooting and Pregnancy

More women are becoming involved in activities that require the use of firearms. Law enforcement, military, and security careers; carrying a firearm for self-protection; and shooting sports require special attention to the needs of pregnant women.

We don't intend this section to constitute medical advice to anyone. It is only a general guide to minimizing the risks of shooting during pregnancy. Any female shooter who is pregnant or plans to become pregnant should consult her doctor about risks that may apply particularly to her. For example, a woman whose checkups during pregnancy have indicated a potentially high risk pregnancy or delivery may be better off avoiding shooting altogether until after the pregnancy.

The fetus is vulnerable to muzzle blast impact noise and to lead exposure. Although the fluid environment surrounding the fetus in the uterus gives some insulation against impact noise, some noise gets through to the fetus. Scientific studies of human subjects have not been conclusive, but some animal studies have demonstrated damage to fetal hearing from intense noise exposure. We cannot be sure that the human fetus is completely immune to hearing damage from shooting noise.

Lead that gets into the mother's body is transferred through the mother's blood to the fetus. It is well established that high lead exposures can cause the baby to have low birth weight or be born prematurely, or can result in miscarriage or stillbirth. Behavioral problems and learning disabilities may also occur in the child exposed to lead before birth.

We have discussed measures to protect the shooter from the known risks of lead and noise, but what about the unborn baby? Even if a pregnant shooter follows these measures faithfully, we must recognize that it is impossible to completely eliminate the risk of exposure to lead and noise. Because of these realities, we recommend that pregnant women refrain from shooting unless absolutely necessary.

Some situations may make it impractical or even hazardous to stop shooting for the duration of pregnancy. A woman's livelihood may depend on her ability to stay proficient with a firearm. Law enforcement officers, security personnel, and firearms instructors are examples where an extended absence from shooting may not be an option. These women can take the following measures to reduce the risk of fetal harm:[7]

- Use lead-free ammunition if possible.

- Shoot on an outdoor range instead of indoors.

- Wear a respirator or mask with a HEPA filter to minimize breathing in lead. Shoot when and where few other people will be shooting, such as non-peak hours at the range.

- Have someone else load and clean your guns.

- Ask your physician to check your blood level of lead. This is a simple blood test that can be done with other routine prenatal laboratory tests.

- Wear layered clothing to help absorb sound.

With this discussion of the risks unique to pregnant women and their unborn babies, we believe most women can make informed decisions about whether they should continue shooting during pregnancy.

The next chapter will address the safety of children in a home with firearms.

Endnotes

1. U.S. Census Bureau web site http://www.census.gov/pubinfo/www/1930facts.html.

2. Kleck G. *Targeting Guns*, 96-97.

3. Kleck G. *Point Blank: Guns and Violence in America*, Aldine de Gruyter, New York 1991: 272.

4. *Ibid.*, 286.

5. American Academy of Otolaryngology-Head and Neck Surgery web site, http://www.entnet.org/healthinfo/hearing/noise_hearing.cfm.

6. *Ibid.*

7. Wrobbel T, "Tips & Tactics: Should the Pregnant Pause?" *Woman's Outlook* 1, no. 3 (March 2003): 12-13.

Chapter Five

Children and Firearms

Most adults are by nature highly protective of their children. The thought of harm coming to our little ones brings many strong emotions, and rightly so. In a home where guns are kept, the responsibility for safety of a child rests solely with the child's parents. Parental responsibility does not end, however, when the child leaves the home. This chapter will discuss how to keep your child safe in the presence of guns, whether inside or outside of the home.

As we know, firearms can be considered a double-edged sword. On the one hand, the head of a household may keep a gun for protection of the family, and yet that same gun places the family at some risk for an accidental child injury or death if the child accesses the gun in an unsafe manner.

Unfortunately, locking your guns away can paradoxically put your family in danger, the exact opposite of your intention. In August 2000, 14-year-old Jessica Carpenter ran from her family's house in Merced, California to get help. Her parents were both away from the house, and a mentally deranged man had broken in and was attacking her younger brother and sisters with a pitchfork. Jessica met two of her sisters outside, and they ran to a neighbor's house.

The sisters begged their neighbor to get his gun and "take care of this guy." But the neighbor refused, instead letting them use his phone to call 911. When the police arrived at the Carpenter home and shot the still-raging killer, they found 7-year-old John and 9-year-old Ashley dead of their wounds.

The horrible irony of this tragedy is that Jessica had been taught how to shoot a gun, and she knew that her father kept a gun at home. She indicated a willingness to use it to stop the murders, but was unable to get to the gun. Her father, fearing prosecution under California's child access prevention law, had secured the gun to keep it away from the children. The children's great-uncle, the Rev. John Hilton, was quoted in the *Fresno Bee* (8/26/2000): "He's [the children's father] more afraid of the law than of somebody coming in for his family. He's scared to death of leaving the gun where the kids could get it because he's afraid of the law. He's scared to teach his children to defend themselves."

The laws of California failed the Carpenter family. The legal climate in that state is such that law-abiding gun owners often feel the sting of the law even more than criminals do. Surely that was the case in Merced.

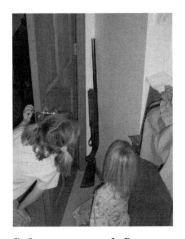

No law can make a family completely safe. When the unthinkable happens, a family must have a plan to meet it, because the unthinkable is not impossible. Risk can come from an outside aggressor, but it can come from within too, in the form of a child who finds a gun and thinks it is a toy. We will describe methods for reducing that risk to a bare minimum.

Safe storage of firearms is very important. A "hidden" shotgun leaning against a wall behind a door is bound to be discovered by curious children.

The Childproof Gun

For many years firearm makers have labored to make their products safer for everyone, and particularly for children. Some of these design features such as external safeties and increasing the force required to pull the trigger have undoubtedly kept some children from harming themselves or others in an accidental shooting.

It is true also that there are many ways to store a gun securely enough that it is quite difficult for a child to get the gun out and unintentionally shoot himself or a playmate. But as parents probably know by observing their own children, no method of gun storage is absolutely childproof. And no design feature can make a gun simultaneously useable and able to resist the motivation and ability of a determined child to explore its workings.

With their remarkably open minds and hunger to learn, children routinely surprise their parents with their evolving abilities to get into danger. Even a 3-year-old can find and get into hiding places that their parents thought secure. As they grow physically and mentally, the challenge of securing guns in the home becomes greater. But parents have no choice other than to meet that challenge.

Banning guns from your own home won't be good enough. Although estimates vary, there are well over 235 million firearms in private hands in the United States. Trying to stop your child from going to a friend's house that contains guns is not reliable, because some owners understandably keep their gun ownership private. The American Academy of Pediatrics, in conjunction with a group called PAX, advises parents to ask the parents of their children's playmates if they have guns in their homes. We do not advise this approach. You are likely to offend gun owners who view their gun ownership as a private matter. Many gun owners, if called by a fellow parent, would deny having guns.

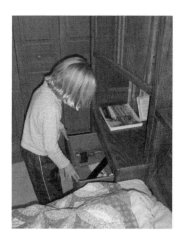

This child is curious about the gun...has she been instructed what to do?

It is highly probable that at least one of your friends or relatives has a gun in their home. People who fear criminal violence enough to own a gun usually fear it enough to keep the gun readily accessible (with variable degrees of locked storage), with ammunition loaded or nearby. This reality cannot be wished away.

Part of being a healthy, normally developing child is a strong and constant tendency to explore. A young couple bringing their first child into the world quickly discovers this marvelous energy, and just as quickly learns the need to protect the child from a long list of household hazards. Swimming pool gate locks, cabinet door locks, and electrical outlet protectors are some of the ways of childproofing the home.

Of course, even with all the known benefits of such simple home safety measures, parents know that they must still always be vigilant. They soon learn that their children, motivated as they are by strong curiosity and enabled by uncanny ability to get into trouble, will defeat many of the devices of adults to protect them. All too soon they will grow tall enough or strong enough to reach that high shelf and find that loaded gun.

Add to this the unrealistic portrayals of guns that children see on television, often at far too tender an age. On TV people get shot all the time, and nothing too bad happens. Certainly there is no hint of wheelchairs and urinary catheters, of paralysis and brain death. Either gunshot victims just go away, or maybe they are healed after a trip to the hospital. And the shooter is often glamorized, or at the very least his act is trivialized in the make-believe world of the little screen. No mention here of remorse, of ruined lives, or of prison.

The forces impelling a child toward disaster with a gun are just as powerful as those that would take him to an early death behind the wheel of a car. The responsible adult will not let his child drive before he is ready. Nor will that parent allow a child to pick up a gun before he is ready. Cars are not made for small children. They are designed for persons old enough to handle the responsibility of piloting two tons of steel and glass at highway speeds.

Likewise, guns are not made for small children. Although gun manufacturers spend considerable money and effort in researching and incorporating safety features, firearms necessarily require a responsible person to be the operator. They always will, despite the understandable wish for a truly childproof gun. In the final analysis, a gun must be reliable. A self-defense gun must be reliable and available. A gun locked in a safe, separate from its ammunition, with a trigger lock in place, may be the closest thing possible to a childproof gun. But it is the farthest thing possible from a useful self-defense tool.

The ingenuity of the average child, coupled with the need for a self-defense firearm that is both reliable and quickly accessible, lead us to an inescapable conclusion—there is no such thing as a childproof gun.

The Gunproof Child

One of us authors (TW) remembers growing up in a farmhouse where a .22 rifle stood in the corner. Although my brothers and I knew where the ammunition was kept, that rifle was never loaded unless our father took us out in the back ten acres for some target practice. It never occurred to us even to touch that gun without asking his permission. We knew what it could do, because when we were no more than eight years old our father had shown us how it could drill a hole through a two-by-four, and how it could make a tin can flip up into the air.

But we knew that if we asked, our dad would take us out to shoot. We had neither fear of that gun nor morbid fascination with it. We learned that it was safe as long as we followed the rules. Our father made sure that my brothers and I were gunproofed at an early age. He taught us by example and demonstration to use guns safely and responsibly. We never had a gun accident at our house, even with three rowdy boys growing up on a farm.

Massad Ayoob discusses the difficulty of childproofing your guns and the consequent necessity of gunproofing your children in his booklet, mentioned above. We highly recommend this little guide, which we list in the Suggested Reading section at the end of this book.

Most important is recognizing the natural curiosity of a child about guns and satisfying that curiosity in a safe way. Be open and honest, because kids can detect evasions and lies. Stonewalling will only whet their curiosity. Be sure your child is old enough to comprehend the destructive force of a gun before you introduce him or her to shooting. There is no hard and fast rule. Some children under age 10 can handle a beginner rifle with confidence and dependable safety.

The winner of the 2003 Steel Challenge World Speed Shooting Championship in California was 15 year-old K.C. Eusebio. As a "child," K.C. wouldn't be able to legally buy his own gun for another six years. But he beat out the top veterans, the legends of handgun speed shooting. In 1999 K.C. was the top pre-teen shooter at the Steel Challenge. The dedication it takes to be that good shows K.C. to be a young man with greater than average maturity.

On the other hand, some adults are too immature to be trusted with a gun. You will know your own child's abilities and be able to task him or her with increasing responsibility according to those abilities.

An excellent age-appropriate program for pre-kindergarten through sixth grade is the National Rifle Association's acclaimed Eddie Eagle GunSafe® Program. In student workbooks, a video, and brochures, mascot Eddie Eagle teaches kids the 4 basic steps to take in case they find a gun:

STOP!

Don't touch.

Leave the area.

Tell an adult.

The children of one of the authors (JW) were taught this program, including its entertaining animated videotape. Several weeks later the children were still chanting and singing the song "Stop, Don't touch, Leave the area, Tell an adult."

The initial steps of "Stop" and "Don't touch" are the most important. These steps remind a child to resist the natural tendency to explore. "Leave the area" allows them to separate and create distance, and "Tell an adult" emphasizes that children should seek a trustworthy and responsible neighbor, relative, or teacher if a parent is not available.

For more information about the Eddie Eagle GunSafe® Program call (800) 231-0752 or visit the NRA's web site at www.nra.org.

In summary, teaching your children safety around guns is based on the same principles as teaching them about other potential hazards. Introduce them to guns at the earliest age that they can understand the cause and effect of guns. Make physical demonstration a part of the instruction when appropriate. Keep the lines of communication open, and be honest about what guns can and cannot do. Defuse the mystery and attraction of firearms by allowing your children to touch and eventually shoot firearms under supervision when you judge them to be mature enough to handle it.

Your child will follow your lead in learning about guns. If you project fear, avoidance, and unrealistic expectations, your child will adopt these dangerous attitudes. They will not serve him or her well in a world where guns in homes are a fact of life.

But if you project confidence, respect for the power of guns, and mastery of the tool, you will give your child the skills to handle firearms confidently and safely, whether he or she chooses eventually to take up shooting or not. To quote from Ayoob, "There is no safety in ignorance."

We have already discussed the need to store firearms safely and the evolution of Rule 5 to recognize this need. In the next chapter we will cover the many options for safe firearm storage in the family setting.

Chapter Six

Storage of Firearms

A firearm must be properly stored if it is to function dependably and not be an unnecessary danger to anyone. Most firearm owners recognize the important responsibility to store their firearms safely, and fortunately there are many ways to do this. The rare accidental shootings involving children and unsuspecting adults are nearly all preventable. Most of these accidents are the results of unauthorized access to the firearm. This chapter will discuss storage of firearms and ammunition, locking devices, and other considerations, with the main goal of keeping your family, friends, neighbors, and loved ones safe.

Choosing a Storage Location

Before choosing a firearm storage method the firearm owner must consider several factors.

How fast do I want to be able to retrieve and use a loaded gun for self-defense in the event of an unexpected threat? There is no absolutely correct answer to this question. Each family must take into account their own philosophy and strategy for dealing with an unexpected and potentially life-threatening encounter with violent criminals. Just as a family should talk about and practice fire drills, there should ideally be discussions about response to potential criminal home invasion, looting, robbery, arson, and other potentially violent situations.

Each family member should be aware of their own individual role and actions, whether it would be running to the family safe room, running away outside, pressing an alarm button, calling 911 for help, or retrieving a firearm or other weapon for self-defense. The decision to rely on a firearm in self-defense is viewed differently by each person, and the entire family should be involved with planning and preparedness.

If the family wants to be able to retrieve a firearm rapidly and use it for self-defense, then the storage of that weapon must easily allow the owner to acquire the firearm, load it with ammunition and use it to protect the family if needed. This same storage method must, however, prevent unauthorized access during the time that no one is using it. This may be a difficult task. We will describe several methods for allowing rapid access while still ensuring security of the home defense firearm.

If the family decides not to have available rapid access to a firearm, other storage options are available. Many experts recommend locking and storing the ammunition in a secure location separate from the guns, thus nearly eliminating the chance of unauthorized access and loading. A variety of very secure gun safes are commercially available, and some are even fire-resistant. Gun safes come with either key locks or combination locks.

How can I store the ammunition so that it will work when needed? High heat and humidity accelerate the breakdown of ammunition components, making it less reliable. Ammunition is best stored in air-tight sealed containers in a cool, dry area of the home, and properly locked or secured so that children and other unauthorized persons cannot get to it. Properly stored ammunition has been known to function perfectly after many decades. However, if the ammunition is carried on one's person daily, such as in law enforcement duty or concealed carry, then that ammunition should be replaced with new ammo every 6 to 12 months or more often. If the ammunition becomes wet or exposed to significant sweat or body oils, then assume that it has been ruined and discard it safely.

Ammunition kept at room temperatures and away from heat sources is not a fire hazard. Even if the home were to catch fire and burn, small quantities of normal rifle and pistol ammunition do not represent a serious threat to firefighters or homeowners attempting to put out the fire. Larger quantities of black powder (used as ammunition in muzzle-loading guns) may be of slightly higher threat. A plastic one-pound container of black powder, however, should not pose a serious threat in a home fire.

If I decide to store my self-defense guns for rapid access, how should I store the ammunition for rapid usage also? If the firearm owner chooses to store the gun and ammunition together for rapid access for self-defense, the ammunition may be stored in one of three general methods: 1) keep it in the original manufacturer's box or lying loose next to the gun as individual cartridges, with the gun unloaded; 2) keep the ammo inside a magazine (or speed loader for revolvers) which is detached from the gun but lies near the unloaded gun; or 3) keep the ammo loaded inside the gun (revolver, semi-automatic, other) ready to fire. There are advantages and disadvantages to each of these storage methods. Choosing the right plan for rapidly deploying a loaded self-defense gun requires weighing these pros and cons, and then making the best decision for your particular situation.

Where should I store my self-defense gun? To answer this question the firearm owner must decide upon a defense plan (see Chapter 9). The defense plan takes into account the potential threats faced by the owner and family, including the layout of the home. The plan should also take into account the location of valuables that the criminal may go after. It should describe the reaction or defense that the family will rely upon if the unexpected potentially violent encounter should occur. If the plan is for everyone to move quickly to a safe room that has a securely lockable sturdy door, with phone access (ideally a mobile phone) and some hard furniture or cover to hide behind, then that safe room would be a good location for storing the firearm.

On the other hand, if there is no plan to stay inside in the case of unexpected break-in (such as if the homeowner lives alone and plans to flee), then the firearm may perhaps best be stored in the area where the homeowner spends the most time when the potential threat is the highest. In this case the gun might be best secured in a locked box in the bedroom, with rapid access to both firearm and ammunition (loaded magazine) during a potential home invasion in the middle of the night. Another example would be a computer programmer who spends much time at his or her home office. This person, who may work late at night, might choose to arrange a secure storage site within easy reach of the computer workstation.

There may be others in a third category who have no intention to store the gun for rapid access for self defense. In order to make it harder for children or others to get to, these gun owners may lock the gun and ammunition away in two different places or safes. These safes may be secured so that no children, adolescents, or others could open them, or painstakingly hidden to make access more difficult for burglars. The disadvantage for the homeowner in this situation is the several minutes it would take to get both the gun and the ammunition separately should he decide to use it for self-defense. A criminal act would likely be over and resolved one way or the other before the homeowner could arm himself.

A homeowner can choose from different degrees of preparedness. The correct choice for storage of a self-defense gun is the location that makes sense for the particular family, meets their unique needs, and prevents unauthorized access.

My spouse has problems with sleepwalking and making decisions at night. Should my spouse have access to our self-defense firearm? One should consider the mental state of adult family members and how they would react if suddenly required to handle the firearm in an emergency. The sleepwalking family member who has been known to do irrational or unpredictable things at night during sleep should certainly not keep a gun in the nightstand or near the bed. This person should not keep the firearm so readily accessible, but instead lock the firearm and ammunition in two different areas. Alternatively, the firearm should be located far enough away that he or she would have awakened completely to a normally functioning mental state before handling a loaded gun.

An elderly parent in the home with dementia such as Alzheimer's disease could possibly shoot a friend or family member because of confusion or mistaken identity. Special precautions should be taken to prevent unauthorized access of a mentally impaired person to self-defense firearms. The same precautions would apply to persons on mind-altering medications or alcohol.

To summarize, the exact storage location and condition of the firearm (degree of readiness) is a personal and family decision that should be made after considering the many factors involved.

What safe storage devices for our guns and ammunition are best for our home? The guiding rule is this—store guns so that they are not accessible to unauthorized persons. The loaded gun simply left in a bedroom drawer is an invitation to disaster. The tallest shelf in the closet will someday be explored by curious little children who grow taller each day, and if that gun becomes a "toy" for that child, the results can be devastating. An 8-year-old boy may be responsible, and he may have mastered proper gun handling techniques. But his 10-year-old cousin may be dangerously unfamiliar with guns. If the 8-year-old brings his cousin in the closet to see Daddy's gun, the cousin may pull the trigger with predictably tragic results. One of the authors has seen that happen twice in the same week in his community. In each of these two separate incidents the victims were brought to his emergency room at a Level I trauma center, both with accidental shotgun wounds to the abdomen. Accidents like this should never happen. They are entirely preventable.

Firearm Locking and Storage Devices

Many gun locking and storage devices are available, and properly used, they are quite effective. However, it is important to remember that any mechanical device can fail. A child's creative imagination and determination may defeat the device, allowing unauthorized access. While no single component of your gun security system is foolproof, a layered system of storage devices, training, and child-proofing can nearly eliminate the chance of tragic accidents.

The household should decide collectively which securing technique is best for them. Keep in mind that many states now require new firearms to be sold with an approved locking device, and so it is possible that the gun may come equipped with one. This may or may not be the best method for your family, but some type of lock or secure storage device should be part of your security plan.

Some state laws also specify which types of gun storage devices may be used. For example, the California Department of Justice lists on its web site the storage devices it considers acceptable.[1] California's child access prevention law provides criminal penalties for failing to reasonably secure a gun from unauthorized access by a child. Always check your state's laws for such legally mandated gun storage requirements. Your state or local gun club can give you advice on how to get this important information.

Firearm Locking Devices

Firearm with built-in lock (combination, key, or magnetic ring)
Some modern firearms are built at the factory or modified to include a lock is that inactivates the gun when locked. This may be a small

3-digit combination wheel that must be properly dialed. Another type of built-in firearm lock requires insertion of a simple key device that may be turned to allow the gun to fire. Revolvers made by the company Taurus International Mfg., Inc. now come with this key-lock feature.

Some experimental models incorporate a finger ring worn by the shooter without which the gun will not fire. Undoubtedly newer techniques will be developed in the future. The gun owner should investigate these devices, discuss them with knowledgeable persons, and try them before purchasing the gun. The advantage is possibly blocking the firing of the gun by unintended persons or children. The disadvantage is the extra time needed to manipulate the locking device, and potential loss of a key or ring that will render the piece of equipment useless in the heat of the attack.

Although integrated locks on firearms provide an extra layer of security against unauthorized use, they also provide an extra barrier for the user to overcome in a rapidly evolving emergency. Fine motor skills are markedly impaired during a life-threatening encounter. Instead of leisurely and smoothly unlocking your gun, you will be trembling with fear. Having to work a tiny lock will present a challenge that could delay your life-saving response to a lethal threat.

Remember too that any lock is just another mechanical device that can fail. Much has been written and said about "personalized guns" with computer chips that allow only the owner to fire them. But a practical and reliable model of such a gun has not been perfected yet. And above all, a self-defense gun must be reliable.

Locking magazine block The locking magazine block is made to fit into the magazine well of a semiautomatic handgun, preventing loading and operation of the gun. It fits into the empty magazine well and is locked in place with a key or combination. The advantage of this type of lock is simplicity and ease of operation. The disadvantage is the time required to inactivate the lock, remove the block, and replace it with a loaded magazine.

External trigger lock Many companies sell a variety of devices that simply clamp onto the trigger area of the gun and lock in place with a key or combination lock. These devices prevent the trigger from being pulled, thus theoretically making it impossible to fire the gun. Ammunition can still be loaded into a gun with a trigger lock in place, but without the trigger pulled the gun is rendered safe. Most are of good design, but the owner should test the device safely to ensure proper function. Guns with trigger locks properly placed have been fired, and manufacturers generally advise unloading the gun before applying the lock. As with other locking devices, there is the disadvantage of a delay in unlocking such a device.

Locking cable The locking cable is a rubber-coated sturdy cable wire that is passed through the chamber, barrel or action of the firearm, and then locked with a key or combination lock. Although the cable could be cut with sufficient force, it is generally very thick and resistant to tampering. This device prevents the gun's action from working, thus rendering it non-loadable and inoperable. Removal of the cable allows immediate use. The advantage is that it is a highly visible method of locking the gun. The cable lock can be removed fairly rapidly with its key or combination. The only disadvantages are fairly minor—the time delay in deploying the gun, and a tendency for dust collection inside its action.

Partial gun locking enclosure The partial gun locking enclosure is a padded hard plastic shell that locks around the gun and prevents access until the key or combination is unlocked. The advantage is that the gun can be fully loaded or magazine inserted (chamber empty), and the gun cannot be fired because the trigger area is fully enclosed. Once unlocked, the gun may be used immediately. The disadvantage is the minor time delay with unlocking.

Unsafe Firearm Storage Devices

- Clothes drawer, top closet shelf, nightstand drawer

- Hollow book, fake clock, and other "hide in plain sight" methods

- Behind doors and other out-of-sight areas

- Unlocked display case or cabinet (glass front, wood, metal)

These methods simply should not be used. Children, however small, always amaze adults with their advanced knowledge and skills. They can gain access to the cleverest hiding places and the highest shelves. Do not trust children to obey your command to "never look there". Do not underestimate their abilities. Even if your

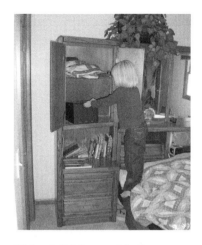

This child is unable to open this electronic gun safe.

children completely obey your directions, you can be assured that their friends will not.

If one of these techniques is used in a household with no children it is important to secure the gun properly should any children or questionable adults enter the home. Take the time to make the firearms safe from curious eyes and fingers. A safer plan is to use a proper locking device or storage device even if no children or unqualified adults live in the household. That way you will already have proper security in place when, for example, neighbor children visit.

Lockable Firearm Storage Devices

Locked gun box with rapid access device (key, touch-pad, electronic access) Both authors especially regard the locked box as one of the top choices for the home defense-minded family. The advantage of this type of storage device is that a fully loaded handgun can be kept close by in a nearly foolproof and childproof locked box. There are several manufacturers and lock types. One of the fastest and most secure boxes has room for one or two handguns and is opened by pressing a combination of 3 sets of numbers. With a little practice one can open the box within 2 seconds. This electronic box has a loud alarm that will sound if more than 5 unauthorized attempts at code breaking occur (i.e. children playing or attempting to open the box).

Another design of locking box uses a Simplex button combination lock. To unlock the box one pushes a brief preset sequence of buttons from a row of five buttons. This allows a knob to be turned, unlocking the box. An advantage of this type of box is that it doesn't rely on electronic circuitry to function. However, it does not have the alarm feature of the electronic device.

Both the manual combination lock and the electronic lock boxes offer a high degree of security and 2-second access to a loaded gun.

Locked gun cabinet or safe These devices offer solid, child-resistant and burglar-resistant storage. They consist of a metal cabinet or box with a heavy-duty combination or key lock. Gun cabinets and safes come in a wide variety of sizes, holding from 1 firearm up to 60. An advantage of some cabinets is that they can be purchased with a fire-resistant ceramic lining as thick as 1 inch or more. This

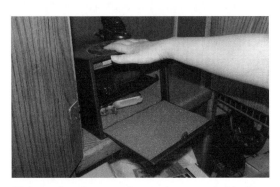

feature reduces greatly the risk of damage from a house fire. Some gun owners and collectors do not want to list their guns or insure their guns with insurance companies, and therefore a fire-resistant gun safe is a good option. The advantages are many, including a cool, dry storage environment for guns and ammunition, fire resistance, burglar resistance, and child resistance. A

This style of gun safe can be opened in less than 2 seconds with the correct pressing of 3 buttons, allowing rapid access to 2 loaded handguns.

disadvantage is the time delay in accessing the gun, since the key or combination must be used to open the gun cabinet. Another disadvantage is the heavy weight of larger ceramic-lined cabinets. They can weigh over 800 pounds and require special equipment to move into the home. Once installed, however, they are well worth the investment of money and work.

Lockable simple portable gun case (fabric, leather, plastic, or aluminum) Gun owners with only a few guns may prefer to use a smaller, portable gun case. Cloth, soft plastic, or leather gun cases can be locked, but are not very child resistant. A hard plastic or aluminum case with a sturdy lock is reasonably child resistant. The advantage of being fairly portable is a mixed blessing, for although they can be easily transported, a thief can just as easily break into the home and steal these cases and their contents. The time delay in unlocking and opening the case is another disadvantage.

Gun automobile lock (law enforcement car locking device) For law enforcement officers, rapid electronic lock release gun storage devices provide a valuable way to secure shotguns and carbine rifles for quick deployment. These devices are generally not available to civilians, as most state laws require transportation of firearms in the back or trunk of the automobile. Since children for the most part are not allowed inside patrol cars, they do not pose a risk of unauthorized access. These locks may allow operation and accidental firing of the shotgun or rifle, and caution should be taken to prevent unauthorized access.

Locked storage closet or room The homeowner may choose simply to place the guns and ammunition in a special locked storage room. A locked closet door or a commercially made metal security door with sturdy frame may be used to deny entry to unauthorized persons and children. A locked storage room may be the best place for a large gun collection or for reloading equipment and shooting gear. The routine locking of such a room must have high priority, as a single episode of leaving the door ajar may result in tragedy.

This concludes the description of the storage devices. The reader should note that the needs and types of gun storage will likely change over the years. Life situations change, and therefore so do the needs for gun storage. You may acquire new guns or get rid of old ones. The 4-year-old child certainly has no business getting access to firearms, but that same child will likely years later become a responsible adolescent. The parents may choose to allow a responsible and properly trained child access to the family's firearms someday. On the other hand, a different family may have a troubled or even suicidal teenager. That family may choose to remove all weapons and guns from the household for a period of time during the crisis. Therefore the firearm owner's choice of storage and access should adapt to changing family circumstances.

How do I transport my gun when traveling? Each state has different legal requirements for traveling with a gun. Making the task more difficult for the interstate traveler is that states frequently change their laws, a fact demonstrated by the current trend toward reciprocity legislation for concealed carry. These laws acknowledge the increasing trend among all but a handful of states to allow concealed carry of firearms for self-protection.

You must find out and abide by the laws of each state through which you will be traveling. The most common method is to transport the gun in a locked gun case (soft or hard), unloaded, with ammunition not readily available. However, concealed carry laws may permit the properly certified person to carry a loaded pistol in a holster. Some laws even specify that a firearm may be placed in the open on the car seat next to the driver. This method, even though technically legal, is probably not wise. Most police officers who might pull you over for speeding would view an openly carried firearm as an immediate threat and would take measures to neutralize that threat. You would very likely find yourself covered with the officer's firearm and handcuffed until the officer assured himself you were just a regular citizen.

In summary, learn the laws, and then decide how best to carry your firearm. Take into account your personal preference, your training, and the presence of children.

Air travel has become much more complicated in recent years because of security measures. Flying with firearms is still possible, although you must learn and follow all the rules. In addition to federal laws and policies of the Transportation Security Administration, each airline has its own procedures and limitations. Check with your airline, and with the state or country you are traveling to. In general, it is fairly easy to travel with firearms.

Make sure the weapon is unloaded. Transport any ammunition in the original box or carton (no loose ammunition or loaded in magazines). Declare the presence of the gun. Federal law requires you to sign and date a small luggage tag that is placed inside your hard-sided, locked suitcase or hard rifle case. Airline personnel may ask you to open your suitcase and prove that the weapon is unloaded. You may need to handle the gun and show that its chamber is empty. If you are asked to do this, make all motions slow and discreet so as not to alarm other travelers. Communicate during this process, and all should go smoothly. Be aware that occasionally guns are stolen during transportation, and make sure your insurance coverage is appropriate. Many countries do not allow weapons of any type to be brought in, and they provide severe penalties for violators. Learn and abide by the rules.

How do I prevent my guns from becoming rusty and unreliable? The first consideration in maintaining a firearm in good working condition is the day-to-day handling and care of the firearm. Always use the correct ammunition as specified by the manufacturer of the gun. Avoid very powerful loads or ammunition hand loaded by inexperienced or careless persons. Properly clean your guns after every shooting session. Keep them adequately lubricated so that metal-on-metal wear does not prematurely shorten the life of the firearm. Most modern guns from reputable manufacturers are designed to last several lifetimes, and shooting up to 100,000 rounds of ammunition from the same gun is not unheard of.

The type of exterior finish on a gun will affect the day-to-day care needed. A blued steel gun finish is sensitive to the salt in perspiration. A gun handled with sweaty hands and put away without cleaning can develop permanent rust marks within 2 or 3 days. On the other hand, a stainless steel weapon, or a hard Parkerized or Teflon finish on the gun will render it more resistant to rusting and general wear-and-tear. This does not mean that the gun can be mistreated or maintained carelessly. Instead, all guns require regular cleaning to ensure reliable function and maximum accuracy.

Follow the manufacturer's directions on how to field strip, clean, lubricate, and reassemble the firearm. A knowledgeable friend or neighbor who can demonstrate the basics of gun maintenance can make the chore easier to learn and more enjoyable.

Inside the gun cabinet or gun storage locker or room there should be placed an electric 110-volt heating rod. These metal rods constantly produce a small amount of heat, keeping the guns and interior of the gun cabinet at a slightly warmer temperature than the surrounding air. When the cabinet or room is opened, the guns are much less likely to accumulate water vapor molecules on the metal surface as cooler and moister air enters the cabinet. This prevents water condensation and the resulting rust and mildew.

Proper storage, cleaning and care of firearms are necessary components of a comprehensive strategy for your family's security program. Just as proper automobile maintenance minimizes the chance of a roadside engine failure or flat tire, proper storage and maintenance of your firearms will ensure that your gun will be ready for emergency use if it is ever needed. These good habits will make your family safe from firearm accidents and external threats alike.

Endnotes

1. California Department of Justice web site, http://ag.ca.gov/firearms/fsd-certlist.php

Chapter Seven

Firearms Training

A responsible gun owner must have a level of competence that will assure safety in handling his or her firearm. That competence is best acquired through training, and thorough training by competent teachers is essential to using a gun for self-defense.

Where can I take a training class? How do I handle my gun safely? How do I shoot it? How do I load it? How do I clear a jammed gun? How do I hit my target in a stressful situation? When can I legally pull the trigger to defend my family and myself? When would I be better off just running away? What should I do if I am forced to shoot in self-defense? What should I do when the police arrive? Will they shoot me if they see me holding a gun? The answers to these important questions should be learned before obtaining a gun for self-defense. We will discuss how to get the proper training you need to answer all these questions and more.

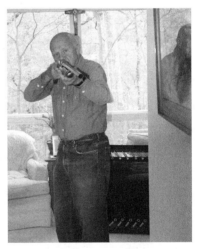

Legendary baseball Hall of Famer Ted Williams is said to have remarked that people always told him that his natural ability and good eyesight were the reasons for his success as a hitter. But, he noted, they never talked about the "practice, practice, practice." It's true that some

Proper firearms training will improve skills and tactics. This photograph shows a homeowner using a shotgun in self-defense, but he is not using cover effectively.

shooters are naturally better than others, but almost everyone can learn formidable firearm skills with proper training. And of course, with practice, practice, practice.

For reasons we will discuss in the chapter on laws and ethics, training in serious self-defense is not a routine thing. We don't learn it in public schools. The principles involved in deciding to learn these skills require the student to confront profoundly serious matters.

It is helpful for the beginner to follow nine steps that will structure these weighty issues in a manageable plan. In following the nine steps the student will become skilled in the use of firearms for self-defense. Properly trained citizens realize that self-defense means far more than buying a gun, loading it, and shooting the bad guy if he comes around. Instead, there is much to be learned, considered, and practiced before one can properly begin to defend oneself and one's family. The student must:

1. Have the motivation to learn about self-defense

2. Learn both armed and unarmed self-defense

3. Learn the basic laws and consequences of self-defense

4. Learn about criminal and self-defense tactics and home security

5. Decide on the proper firearms for you and your family

6. Choose and complete a firearm safety course, including firing range practice

7. Choose and complete a self-defense course (e.g., tactics or combat shooting)

8. Develop and practice personalized self-defense and home defense strategies

9. Practice, modify and improve skills and tactics as needed. Continue to learn.

These nine steps can be learned in a matter of weeks or over a few years. As in life itself, there should be a gradual progression of skills and knowledge that improves over the years. Learning opportunities will be determined by your available time and resources. Good training facilities may be available locally, or their location may require some travel and hotel arrangements. The goal is to become an accomplished marksman with the skills to shoot accurately under stress. The ultimate test of those skills—confronting a threat of deadly force—is a test that the wise citizen should never want to take. But if that test is ever thrust upon the citizen, that properly trained person would have what it takes to survive with his or her family intact.

Before you can keep your family safe you must be sure that they don't hurt themselves or others unintentionally by mishandling a firearm. Family members should become familiar with firearms, learning about them and handling them in a safe environment and then practicing until their skills are solid. Then they should go to the shooting range every three to six months or more often if possible, to maintain skill levels. Marksmanship skills deteriorate with time, and only by regular practice can one be assured of not only of maintaining basic firearms skills, but also make sure that the weapon itself is reliable and functioning properly.

So let's review the Nine Step Process for becoming competent in self-defense.

1. Have the motivation to learn about self-defense. Each reader has his or her own unique experiences and ideas about self-defense. Therefore the motivation towards protecting self and family will vary considerably. Some citizens choose not to own firearms, and may therefore keep a baseball bat, fire poker, or other weapon nearby for use "just in case". Others may adopt the ostrich method of self and family defense, and simply hope or pray that a deadly threat never happens. These people have neither the plan nor the means for effective self-defense. Depending on luck, they are at the mercy of the criminals who select them as victims.

At the other end of the spectrum is the gun enthusiast who has taken multiple combat gun courses, owns 10 pistols, and keeps 3 loaded guns in his home and car at all times. Each of these people has a different level of motivation to seek training. Motivation must come from within, or as a response to acquired information or threats. Conservative estimates suggest that there are well over 2 million occurrences of self-defense with guns in the United States each year. Armed self-defense usually results in successfully repelling or stopping violent crime from occurring, and most of the time not a single shot is fired. The simple presence of a firearm in the hands of a determined and obviously competent defender is enough to make most violent criminals hastily reconsider their choice of victim. Firearms have stopped many crimes and will continue to do so for those who choose this effective means of self-defense.

2. Learn both armed and unarmed self-defense. The serious student of self-defense must learn unarmed self-defense skills in addition to firearm skills. The reason is simple. Not every criminal threat should be met with the lethal force possible with a firearm. An example would be the bully who confronts you and your family on the street. Attempting to flee is a worthy idea, but may not be possible if your family includes little children. If the bully shoves and curses you, but does not threaten your life or show a weapon, your response of drawing a gun would be inappropriate and unlawful in most circumstances. Many other possible situations may simply require blocking and evasion self-defense techniques to resolve the conflict.

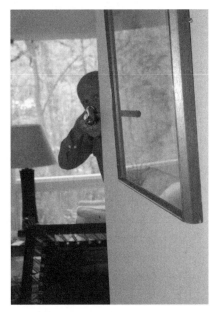

Unarmed self-defense techniques include proper defensive stance, defensive blocking moves, defensive tactics (when to run and when to stay and fight), disarming techniques, psychological techniques, strikes with hand, elbow, feet, and knees, and fighting on the ground.

Good tactics save lives. This photo demonstrates a good firing position of a homeowner who is hiding most of his body behind cover.

Many self-defense experts recommend an intermediate defense weapon such as pepper spray, also known as OC spray (oleoresin capsicum). The use of this weapon will not be discussed in detail, other than pointing out that in some situations pepper spray may be an ideal defensive tool. Learn about it during your defensive training schools. There are advantages and disadvantages of every technique.

Basic firearm understanding can be initiated by simply reading a few books. Learn about the parts of guns, and how they work. This should be done before going to the first classroom session, and will provide a solid foundation for future firearms education.

The healing arts and the martial arts may be a world apart in ordinary thinking, but they are parallel in several senses. In both, the less intervention needed, the better. Both disciplines involve strategy in dealing with disease or conflict, and in both, knowledge of the problem provides the key to the solution. A good defender will know the enemy, and with knowledge of common criminal behaviors will be able to choose and apply a suitable defense technique.

3. Learn the basic laws and consequences of self-defense. Each state has slightly different versions of the law regarding self-defense, property defense, and use of lethal force by civilians. Much of this may be learned in the classroom, but several excellent books explain the laws, outcomes, and consequences of using deadly force. We list some of these references in a section at the end of this book. The wise defender will know the legal boundaries of armed and unarmed self-defense, and will know when and when not to use them.

If you ever pull the trigger and use deadly force to stop a violent criminal, the full ramifications and legal consequences should be fully known beforehand. Proper knowledge will underline how very important it is to use lethal force only as a final option after exhausting all other reasonable alternatives for resolving the conflict.

4. Learn about criminal and self-defense tactics and home security. Know the enemy. What threats could you and your family face? What security problems should you reasonably make plans to deal with? What do you do when you hear that bump in the night downstairs? What is the best response?

Defending yourself may be entirely different from defending the whole family, who may not have the option of running away or defending themselves. As we discussed in the previous chapter, home security is composed of several layers of deterrence and warning systems. Books and courses teach tactics for home defense, and these should be studied and discussed with instructors.

What about self-defense while traveling in a car or camper? What laws affect your response? Your state or local laws controlling vehicle firearm transport and access may differ from the laws governing home firearm storage and access. It will be your job in this step to become familiar with those laws.

5. *Decide on the proper firearms for you and your family.* If you have researched this topic well and discussed it with friends whose knowledge you respect, then make the decision to buy the firearms that best meet your needs. You may choose to make an actual purchase after the start of or completion of firearm safety and defense instruction classes. If uncertain, then proceed to steps 6 and 7 before buying a gun. Each family's situation will dictate the best method of self-defense with a firearm. For example, if the family decides upon having a safe room to retreat to in case of criminal violence, the 120-pound mother may wish to have an easy-to-handle semi-automatic

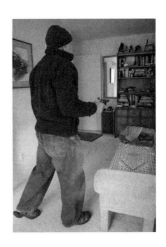

The criminal has broken into a home and is armed with a handgun. Will you know how to defend your family if this happens in your home?

20-gauge shotgun to protect her family, instead of a powerful handgun with recoil too hard to control. On the other hand, many women can handle quite powerful firearms, while some men may be better off with a less powerful gun that they can more accurately shoot. The person who must conduct business in dangerous parts of a city may choose a concealable handgun, get a concealed carry license, and use a compact self-defense handgun as part of a home defense strategy as well.

6. *Choose and complete a firearm safety course, including firing range practice.* Few of us are fortunate enough to have friends or associates who can safely and expertly instruct them in firearm safety. Most citizens should seek and complete a firearms safety course that focuses on the type of gun they plan to buy and use. The five basic safety rules should be learned and practiced until they are second nature. The class should ideally include on-range firing of the individual student's gun with close one-on-one supervision to prevent accidents and teach efficiently.

You should do considerable practice with actual self-defense ammunition, which is more powerful and therefore causes greater felt recoil. Care should be taken to avoid the bad habits of flinching or jerking the trigger. Both result in missing the target. Good marksmanship habits should be learned and practiced. A good instructor will teach you the proper stance or other position, the right grip on the firearm, how to line up the sights, how to place the sights on your target, and how to pull the trigger smoothly. All these steps are essential to putting your bullet exactly where you want it to go. Willing students learn quickly, and watching your accuracy improve is exciting. Practicing your new skills makes perfect. And remember, safety should always be the number one priority.

7. *Choose and complete a self-defense course (e.g., tactics or defensive shooting).* Once the new shooter has learned basic gun handling and safety, and has the skill to put a bullet on target consistently, it is time to learn the topics of tactics and defensive shooting. What are tactics? Simply put, tactics is the art or skill of using available means to reach an end, of disposing and maneuvering forces in combat. Before getting a gun and engaging in a life or death situation, students should learn the tactical decision-making skills necessary to deal with a criminal violent attack. Learn how to outmaneuver and outsmart a criminal adversary. The best way to do this is to attend a reputable school of defensive shooting and tactics. At such a course, the student learns to draw rapidly and shoot accurately under conditions designed to simulate the stress of fighting. The combat shooting student will engage targets while moving out of the line of attack, using cover, running, backing up, and walking forward. Some drills are conducted in realistic

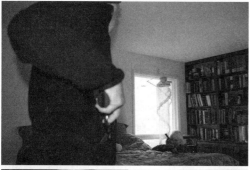

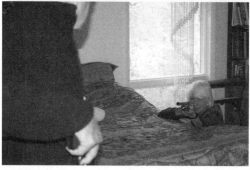

This burgler has just kicked in the bedroom door and is threatening the woman hiding in her safe room. She has called 911 already and is now faced with a stranger who is pulling something out of his pocket. What is the correct response?

low-light or nighttime conditions, since most civilian self-defense shootings occur under these conditions.

Tactics taught in typical classes include guidelines for the use of force, retreating to a safe room, "pie-ing" a room (slowly rounding a corner looking for the bad guy), using a flashlight to assist when shooting in dark conditions, learning the few times when you should clear a house and the more common scenario of when not to, and many other topics. You will learn how a criminal sizes up a potential victim and approaches with a common question, such as asking you the time of day. Learn simple facts such the number one sign that you are about to be attacked or robbed—the criminal will repeat your command back you. "What, you want me to stop and stay away? Hey, I ain't gonna hurt you, I just want to know what time it is." His talking is a technique of distracting your attention as he closes the distance between himself and you, his selected victim.

You will discover that most home burglaries involve two or more criminals, so if you hear and hold a burglar at gunpoint waiting for the police, most of the time there is another burglar outside in a get-away car, or worse, inside your home hiding and waiting. Knowing this and other facts will give the defender an edge when faced with violence. Overall, attending a tactics and combat shooting course will give additional knowledge and skills that will increase the confidence and ability of the gun owner. You will learn valuable facts and methods that may save your life and keep your family safer.

8. *Develop and practice personalized self-defense and home defense strategies.* Once your foundation of defense knowledge and ability is solid, you can build on your knowledge. This stage of self-defense education involves applying your new skills to your own family's situation. What are the potential threats, how can the threats be detected early, how should the family react, what signal or alarm will be sounded, where should family members go, and who should attempt to confront or run from the violent attacker? Your family can develop a personalized self-defense strategy that takes into consideration the many factors unique to your family, as we have mentioned previously. Such a plan may be complex, but will be the best insurance policy in the rare case of the always-unexpected home invasion or violent attack.

9. *Practice, modify and improve skills and tactics as needed.* Continue to learn. Life is about learning, and the passing of time

will present still more opportunities for learning. You may meet new teachers or students with different viewpoints, and you can add their lessons to your skill set. There is no substitute for routine practice, and realistic training can sharpen the abilities and skills of the shooter. Many competitive shooting events scattered across the country offer opportunities to mingle with other like-minded citizens interested in serious methods of self-preservation, perfection of skills, and learning. The International Defensive Pistol Association (www.idpa.com) offers competitive events with handguns meant for self-defense. Typical matches include timed scenarios or "stages" requiring the shooter to use his or her skills in shooting from behind cover, from sitting or prone positions, and reloading, all the time observing safety rules.

Your local gun club may sponsor other similar shooting events, all conducted in the spirit of friendly competition. Regular shooters at these fun events are usually eager to welcome newcomers and help them get started.

Resources for Firearm Training

Where can I get firearms training? At the end of this chapter we will list some nationally recognized modern shooting schools. This list reflects the authors' knowledge and experience only, and it is by no means a complete listing of good schools. To supplement this list, the student should ask at a local gun store the names of regional or local shooting classes that may be quite acceptable and much closer to home.

What skills will I need to learn during firearms training? A beginning course will usually start with the assumption that you know how your gun works and that you know the fundamentals of gun safety. This book, your owner's manual, and the range experience we have recommended will provide you with those skills.

In class you will learn how to position your body (stance), grip, sight alignment, sight picture, and trigger control. Becoming familiar with the operation of safeties on your gun and clearing weapon stoppages and malfunctions will require you to perform repeated drills to acquire the "muscle memory" necessary to do these tasks under stress.

You will cover the variety of holsters, drawing from holsters, drawing from concealed cover (under a coat, jacket, purse, shoulder or ankle holster), one-handed and two-handed shooting styles, recoil management, rapid reloading, use of cover and concealment, and up close and far away shooting techniques. Care, maintenance, and storage of firearms are usually a part of beginning courses.

More advanced courses would include shooting on the move (moving toward, away from, or lateral to a threat), vocalizing while engaging targets, combining hand-to-hand combat blocking skills with drawing and shooting up close, shooting with the non-dominant or weak hand, shooting from prone, kneeling, and other positions; engaging multiple targets, weapon recognition, and yelling commands for threat management.

What skills should I practice when I go to the shooting range? Formal courses will introduce you to all the skills we have mentioned. But this is only a beginning. Mastering and refining those skills will require some range time.

With a partner timing you, practice shortening your draw-and-shoot time. Start slowly and deliberately, getting your hands and eyes familiar with the right moves before trying for a faster time. In practicing your drawing and firing, remember the slogan "Slow is smooth; smooth is fast." Timing your performance has the added benefit of inducing a sense of competitiveness or urgency that simulates, if only in greatly diluted form, the stress of a lethal encounter.

How do I learn and practice my unarmed self-defense skills? Many communities have schools that teach unarmed defensive skills. Since schools vary considerably in their approaches and techniques, we suggest that the student discuss the school's particular skills and philosophies with its teachers, looking for a match of your objectives with those of the school. A sparring partner who wears protective shock-absorbing gear will be a great help. Only with proper training and appropriate supervision should you try to master advanced unarmed combat skills. The need to practice regularly applies as much to unarmed combat techniques as it does to shooting.

How can I integrate my unarmed self-defense skills with techniques using weapons such as a folding knife, pepper spray, and firearm? Schools that teach these methods are rare and certainly not for everyone. But such instruction is available for civilians who desire it. Some novices find they have a strong interest in such advanced proficiency. They should not be afraid to pursue it.

Do any schools offer classes in home defense, car defense, and concealed carry tactics?

As more states pass laws allowing licensed carry of concealed self-defense guns, schools are offering instruction in these types of tactics. Most citizens in reasonably good physical condition and mental health and with no criminal record can enroll in any number of classes. The degree of proficiency you attain is limited only by your time and willingness to learn.

List of schools and training resources

No list would be complete without mentioning the oldest civilian firearm training organization in America—the National Rifle Association (NRA). The NRA was started just after the Civil War by Union generals who wanted to promote and encourage rifle shooting. Dissatisfied with the marksmanship skills of their troops, they set out to improve those skills among the population from which they recruited.

Today the NRA's Training Department offers training from the beginner level up through a nationwide network of nearly 50,000 instructors, coaches, and training counselors. You can find in most communities at least one NRA-certified instructor. A phone call to the NRA's headquarters in Fairfax, Virginia will get you started. Or better yet, become an NRA member and get regular updates on training and other activities in your area.

National Rifle Association of America

11250 Waples Mill Road

Fairfax, VA 22030-9400

(703) 267-1000

(703) 267-1500 (Education and Training)

www.nra.org

We list the other training institutions in alphabetical order with their mailing addresses, telephone numbers, and web sites. This list is by no means complete, and other schools not listed may be quite satisfactory. We encourage our readers to fully explore and research several firearms training centers before selecting one.

American Small Arms Academy

P.O. Box 12111 / Prescott, AZ 86304

(928) 778-5623 / www.chucktaylorasaa.com

Gunsite Academy

2900 W. Gunsite Road/ Paulden, AZ 86334-4301

(928) 636-4565 / www.GunCite.com

InSights Training Center

P.O. Box 3585 / Bellevue, WA 98009

(425) 827-2552 / www.insightstraining.com

Lethal Force Institute

P.O. Box 824 / Fairfield, CT

(203) 261-8719 / www.defenseassociates.com

SIG SAUER Academy

233 Exeter Road / P.O. Box 903 / Epping, NH 03042

(603) 679-2003 / www.sigsaueracademy.com

Tactical Firearms Training Team

16835 Algonquin Street, Suite 120 / Huntington Beach, CA 92649

(714) 206-5168 / www.tftt.com

Thunder Ranch

96747 Hwy 140 East / Lakeview, Oregon 97630

(541)-947-4104 / www.thunderranchinc.com

U.S. Training Center Moyock

P.O. Box 1029 / Moyock, NC 27958

(252) 435-2488 / www.ustraining.com

U.S. Training Center also has locations in Illinois and California.

Chapter Eight

Ethics and Laws of Self Defense

This chapter may make some readers uncomfortable. We will discuss a fundamental problem that has confronted humanity since its beginnings—the sad fact that some human beings prey on the innocent. Even before the Christian era philosophers grappled with this problem. Our state and federal lawmakers still do today. The 17th century English philosopher Thomas Hobbes described the condition of confusion, uncertainty, and violence that existed prior to government. Hobbes called this pre-civilized condition the "state of nature." In the state of nature, life was "solitary, poor, nasty, brutish, and short." His solution was a government whose job was, among other things, to enforce laws and keep the peace.

But we know that the government is frequently unable to enforce those laws. The job of police is mostly to take a report and try to catch criminals after a crime has occurred, not before. We also know that the peace is regularly disturbed in violation of our social contract, and innocent people suffer because of it. The police cannot be everywhere, on every street corner, in every dark alley, and in every home.

While this book is not intended as a philosophy text, we believe it is important that our readers know that a desire to gain a working knowledge of self-defense is not being unduly fearful. In the midst of the most advanced civilization ever known, with a level of health and well being unprecedented in history, we still have daily reminders of how thin the veneer of civilization can be.

Any large-scale catastrophe—a hurricane, riot, pandemic, nuclear attack, or an attack with chemical or biological weapons—can create the conditions for social breakdown. Americans saw on September 11, 2001 how easily such attacks can be carried out. Public health authorities have been openly concerned about a pandemic of influenza such as avian influenza or "bird flu." In those circumstances supply lines for water, food, shelter, and lifesaving medication will be disrupted to some extent. History shows that the only way to protect home supplies of these essentials from criminals is with a resolute and armed homeowner.

Within the last two decades three American disasters showed again how stripping away the bonds of social order, even temporarily, brings life-threatening hazards. In April 1992 the Los Angeles riots, brought on by a court verdict in the Rodney King case, turned a large swath of Los Angeles into a nightmare of violence and destruction. Many of the looters and assailants were found to be ordinary criminals taking advantage of the chaos.

In Koreatown, just blocks north of the epicenter of rioting in south central Los Angeles, owners of businesses and homes protected themselves with firearms. The violent mobs bypassed them for easier prey.

Four months after the Los Angeles riots, Hurricane Andrew roared through Dade County, Florida, leaving a quarter million people homeless. Many homeowners stayed with the roofless ruins of what once had been their homes, warning that they would shoot looters.

And in late August 2005, Gulf Coast residents learned the need for armed self-defense. Hurricane Katrina was one of the most devastating tropical storms in the last century, causing at least 1,330 deaths, thousands of injuries, and nearly $100 billion of property damage. In the aftermath, residents quickly found they had to depend on themselves for personal and home security.

New Orleans police were vastly overwhelmed by the general disorder, and some abandoned their posts or even joined in the looting. In the wrecked and deserted Garden District, residents Charlie Hackett and John Carolan established an armed neighborhood watch. According to a September 5, 2005 Fox News report, "Looters smashed windows and ransacked a discount store and a drugstore a few streets over. Three men came to Carolan's house asking about his generator and brandished a machete. He showed them his gun and they left."[1]

All of these disasters were characterized by profound disorganization, fear, and the inevitable appearance of violent criminals. Assaults, robberies, rapes, and murders increased, unchecked by an effective police presence. They also had in common another characteristic—the police were either ineffective in stopping the violence or they were nowhere to be found. Looters and violent opportunists under normal conditions are constrained by a fear of the law. When life is good and business proceeds as usual we tend not to remember that such people even exist. We would rather not think of them. Our human tendency is to deny that anyone would take advantage of innocent people when we all should be pulling together to recover from a natural disaster.

The people of Los Angeles, south Florida, and the Gulf Coast learned an age-old lesson, known to the ancient Greeks and repeated endlessly over the ages. They learned that when civilization's limits on humankind's worst impulses are even temporarily removed, the criminal subculture will dependably assert itself. The strong will seek out the weak as prey. The average criminal is deterred from committing a crime by the fear of being shot or caught by police. When the police are unable to restrain them with this threat, as is so often the case in large-scale disasters, each citizen must protect his own life and property.

The local authorities in New Orleans reacted improperly by ordering the confiscation of firearms from flood victims, often in their own homes at gunpoint. A subsequent court ruling found these seizures illegal, and Mayor Nagin was ordered to return the seized firearms to their rightful owners. Ten months after Hurricane Katrina, Louisiana Governor Kathleen Blanco signed into law the Emergency Powers Protection Act, which aims at preventing similar seizures of citizens' firearms by local governments.

The illegal firearm confiscations by local government in the disorganization following Katrina were hopefully an aberration that will not happen again. In fact, most front-line police officers understand all too well the ultimately personal nature of a citizen's responsibility to provide his own family's security during such massive disasters as Katrina.

The president of the Illinois Tactical Officers Association, police chief Jeff Chudwin, was in New Orleans in the aftermath of Katrina. Chief Chudwin, who is also an attorney, joined a volunteer group of tactical police officers detailed to downtown New Orleans. Their job was to provide security and assist in the search for victims. After that experience he observed "The greatest responsibility of government is to ensure the safety of the public. When government cannot do so because of calamity and disaster, the citizen must bear this burden. Ultimately we are individually responsible for the protection and welfare of our families and selves."[2]

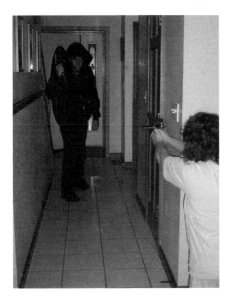

"Ultimately we are individually responsible for the protection and welfare of our families and ourselves." - Chief of Police Jeff Chudwin

Anyone who reads the papers or watches television news knows that violent crime exists even in the absence of natural or man-made disasters. The state of nature can exist for a few minutes in a dark alley, or in a home invaded by violent career criminals. But in those lonely and terrifying moments, a resolute and righteous defender can enforce the laws. In fact, he or she has the right to stop a violent attacker by any means necessary to preserve life and limb.

The Natural Right of Self Defense

Philosophers since ancient times have recognized the fault in human nature that makes some people seek to victimize others. They wrote about the necessity of a legal basis for self-defense. The Roman statesman and writer Marcus Tullius Cicero, who died in 43 B.C., wrote this timeless observation about self-defense:

Civilized people are taught by logic, barbarians by necessity, communities by tradition; and the lesson is inculcated even in wild beasts by nature itself. They learn that they have to defend their own bodies and persons and lives from violence of any and every kind by all the means within their power.[3]

Cicero's wise commentary came from his own hard experience during the tumultuous decline of the Roman Empire. His writings were part of the body of classical works that centuries later guided the English philosophers and legal scholars. These men were in turn the teachers of America's founders. The notions of private property, individual rights, and the right of self-defense—rights we take for granted in 21st century America—all emerged from this philosophical tradition.

One of those English philosophers was John Locke, whose 1698 classic *Two Treatises of Government* influenced America's founders. Locke challenged the ancient doctrines of slavery and the divine right of kings. In the second treatise he explains under which circumstances a person may use lethal force to defend himself.

If a man with a sword in his hand demands my purse on the highway, Locke reasons, when perhaps I don't even have 12 pennies in my pocket, this man I may lawfully kill. But if I deliver to another man 100 pounds of my money to hold only temporarily, and he draws his sword to defend his wrongful possession of it by force, I cannot lawfully even hurt this man, much less kill him.

Locke goes on to explain why natural law allows him to use lethal force in the former instance, when the armed robber may take only pennies from him; but not in the second, when the wrongdoer takes far more of his money. In the second case, the man who took his money and refused to give it back only threatened lethal force when the rightful owner tried to take it back. There was no immediate and unavoidable threat to the owner's life, and "the owner had the benefit of appealing to the law, and have reparation for my 100 pounds that way."

But in the first case the highwayman threatened not only to take his few pennies, but also his life. The assailant made this a clearly lethal threat with sword in hand. Locke concludes the lesson with a self-evident truth:

> The reason whereof is plain: because the one using force, which threatened my life, I could not have time to appeal to

the law to secure it. And when it [my life] was gone, 'twas too late to appeal. The law could not restore life to my dead carcass. The loss was irreparable; which to prevent, the Law of Nature gave me a right to destroy him who had put himself into a state of war with me, and threatened my destruction.[4]

To understand how profound this proposition is we must remember the character of Locke's world. Even though the monarchy no longer wielded unlimited power in 17th century England, it still retained tremendous political authority. There was no lobbying legislators, no arguing policy in the local newspaper, and no city hall debates with concerned citizens voicing their preferences. Life and death decisions were made by the king and his men, and implemented by force. Slavery was widespread and accepted. Throughout most of the world, a person's position and opportunities in life were determined entirely by the family or tribe he or she happened to be born into.

The notion that a person's body and even his home were his own was a novel concept, only then beginning to take hold. The natural right of self-defense was revived as England's political system placed increasing value on the individual, a concept that would soon receive its classic expression in the American Declaration of Independence.

Three centuries later in America, Locke's lesson has been incorporated into the laws of most states. Although state laws on self-defense vary, the guiding principle for using lethal force in self-defense is this: *Lethal force may be used only when undertaken to escape imminent and unavoidable danger of death or grave bodily harm.*[5]

This short statement contains a world of empowerment—the right under law to use force capable of killing a person. It also very severely limits the circumstances under which such overwhelming and decisive force may be used. Although many Americans know that they are somehow authorized under law to shoot someone who is trying to kill them, most have no idea of the profound personal and legal consequences of doing so.

Natural Law and Criminal Law

We have shown that the fundamental principle of the right to self-defense is many centuries old. It has been adopted, reinterpreted, and in some cases significantly changed by centuries of court decisions and legislative modifications.

The result in 21st century America is a bewildering variety of exceptions and contingencies on the law as it is applied in courtrooms every day across the country. Under the U.S. constitution, the states have jurisdiction over most criminal matters. This includes the laws relating to armed self-defense. These statutes are different for every one of the 50 states, and within a state the law is often applied differently from one jurisdiction to another.

For these reasons, a full discussion of practical law considerations of armed self-defense is well beyond the scope of this book. Still, it is vital for every person considering having a gun for self-defense to learn the laws in his or her own state and how local courts apply them. State firearm owners' associations are an excellent place to start learning about the laws in your area. These groups may publish guides for gun owners or be able to guide you to books or classes on armed self-defense law.

Understanding the conditions under which your community allows lethal force is absolutely essential. If you violate any part of the law through ignorance of its provisions, you can and will be prosecuted. You will find that the court considers you to be the criminal, with all the serious trouble that entails. You will be tried and convicted, unless you can convince a jury that your actions were justified.

Even if you did follow the letter and spirit of the law in using lethal force, you are still likely to be arrested. Police and prosecutors handle lethal force encounters in a strictly specified way. If they have any doubts at all about who is at fault, they will arrest all involved parties and hold them in jail until they know whom to charge.

Nor is there any guarantee that a jury will see the case the same way you saw it when death stared you in the face. But juries are still the best assurance of fair consideration by people who are likely to share your values. For example, if you live in a conservative rural or suburban area where people uphold the right of self-defense, a jury will likely be composed of people who will not convict you if you reasonably followed the law.

Contrast that scenario with the nightmare recently suffered by Brooklyn father Ronald Dixon. Dixon shot a burglar who had broken into his home and was going through dresser drawers in Dixon's two-year-old son's bedroom. The burglar, who had a 14-page rap sheet for burglary and larceny, survived.

But Dixon, a Navy veteran with no criminal record, was jailed and charged with misdemeanor gun possession. The Brooklyn district attorney vowed to send him to Riker's Island, the same prison the burglar would go to. Dixon had legally purchased the handgun in Florida and was in the process of getting a permit to own it through New York's notoriously complicated approval process. The assault on his home occurred before New York officials got around to issuing his license, so technically Dixon possessed his gun illegally.

Ironically the district attorney acknowledged that Dixon's use of lethal force was justified, but still intended to ruin his career and damage his life by imprisoning him on the illegal possession charge. The D.A. did not explain how Dixon could have prevented rape or death in his home that morning without using his illegal gun. Dixon finally had to plead guilty to a reduced charge of disorderly conduct and accept a sentence of 3 days in jail. Only a nationwide outcry over the injustice of his case prevented a harsher sentence.

Such is the capriciousness of the law. Never assume that because you followed the law as you understand it that a jury will see it the same way. Even two different juries may apply the law to the facts in a case in ways that produce completely different verdicts. As the Dixon case shows, states and localities vary widely in how they view gun ownership. Owning a gun in New York City, to say nothing of using it in self-defense, is fraught with legal peril not seen in most other areas of the country. Let the gun owner beware.

Criminal charges are not the only legal risk an armed defender faces. A violent criminal can and will sue you for any injuries you inflict on him in the course of defending your life from his attack. Or his survivors will sue you, if he dies. Prepare to defend yourself from this third assault, this time on your family's finances. That a career criminal could use the law to harm you and your family again is grotesquely unfair, but it is the law. Even if the judge throws the case out of court with a summary judgment, you will still have to pay attorney fees. These could easily run into tens of thousands of dollars.

The legal problems an armed defender will encounter are daunting. They reflect the seriousness with which the law views lethal force in a citizen's hands. They can be considered hurdles you must jump in order to survive intact after using that most final sanction, the taking of a human life.

Encouraging changes in state law are happening as the result of such injustices as Ronald Dixon endured. In the last few years over 20 states have passed "castle doctrine laws." These laws remove any duty to retreat if you are attacked in any place where you have a right to be. You are allowed to stand your ground and meet deadly force with deadly force if you reasonably believe your life or limb is in danger. The castle doctrine law also provides that a righteous armed defender can be neither prosecuted by the government nor sued by his assailant.

More states are considering passing castle doctrine laws. This trend, if it continues throughout the states, should go a long way toward restoring the natural right of self-defense. But much work remains before the legal perils of armed self-defense are removed, and it remains to be seen how these new laws will be applied by the courts. For now, we must accept that after one survives the criminal assault, the next step is to survive the legal assault.

The Question

Taking the life of another human being is a violently unnatural act. It goes against much that we learn in our families, communities, churches, and schools. Nevertheless, the law clearly allows us to use lethal force to prevent killing or crippling injury of ourselves or those under our protection.

Religious authorities also acknowledge a basis in natural law for self-defense. The Catholic Church states this principle formally in its *Catechism* (Second Edition) with a discussion of the Fifth Commandment, "Thou shalt not kill." The *Catechism* reads "Legitimate defense can be not only a right but a grave duty for one who is responsible for the lives of others. The defense of the common good requires that an unjust aggressor be rendered unable to cause harm" and "Love toward oneself remains a fundamental principle of morality. Therefore it is legitimate to insist on respect for one's own right to life. Someone who defends his life is not guilty of murder even if he is forced to deal his aggressor a lethal blow."

But few people know how or when they are allowed to exercise the awful power that is sufficient to end a life. The reason we don't have courses in high school or college about the proper use of deadly force is that in spite of the natural law tradition of self-protection, we are still ambivalent about taking human life.

People naturally use the common psychological defense mechanism of denial to put this subject out of their minds. Any consideration of life and death matters is uncomfortable, and the best way to avoid that discomfort is to downplay its importance. We use denial to discount the serious possibility that we could die any day in an auto accident, or in a violent encounter on the street.

Denial is a useful psychological mechanism when it allows us to get through a day without being paralyzed by fear or doubt. But when it keeps us from clearly assessing a threat, it makes us vulnerable. What is the threat to you and your family? Is it realistic to believe that you could be victimized by a violent criminal? What could happen in a worst-case scenario to you or the people you love and are obliged to protect?

You probably already know in a general way how likely it is that your family will be threatened by violent crime. If you live in a dangerous neighborhood with a high crime rate, it will be no secret to you. Likewise, if you are lucky enough to have a home in a fairly safe area, with good police patrols and law-abiding neighbors, your risk is likely quite low.

But how much risk is too much? Is it possible to lower your risk even further than it may already be? Or are there special high-risk situations in your otherwise safe life, such as driving through a bad part of town on the way to work, or being the proprietor of a business with late hours?

Many people don't even ask these questions because they are too uncomfortable to think about. Since you are reading this book, it is likely that they have crossed your mind. If so, you have addressed a reality that confronts us all, whether we choose to recognize it or deny it. We are all, to varying degrees, at risk for victimization by violent criminals. This is as true as the fact that we are all at risk for early death from sickness or injury. Practical-minded people prepare for these realities of life by making arrangements in advance. They take out life or disability insurance. They avoid drinking while driving, and they wear their seat belts. They consider how their families would manage if they were suddenly gone, and they take measures to provide for them.

Assessing your risk of crime victimization and making arrangements in advance is essentially the same. By acknowledging that the risk exists, then determining how great it is for you and your family, you can take logical steps to reduce it. Knowing your family will be provided for financially if you die is a great comfort. Likewise, knowing you have taken all possible steps to protect them from harm gives confidence and peace of mind.

Of all the questions that one must ask in assessing risk of violent crime and your response to it, one is all-important. Everyone considering the use of a firearm for personal protection must ask himself or herself *"Am I willing to kill another human being?"* The natural law and criminal law say you are allowed to use deadly force in order to save your own life. But does your heart agree?

Lt. Col. David Grossman, the military scientist and author, describes "a powerful, innate human resistance toward killing one's own species."[6] He describes how even military training often fails to erase this strong natural aversion to killing. If regimented military training fails to overcome it, how must the average civilian feel when confronted with this awful possibility?

Our purpose in presenting such a bleak picture of armed self-defense is not to discourage our readers. On the contrary, we want them to know they have an indisputable legal and moral basis for self-protection. But we also feel obliged to tell the truth as we know it. The time to discover and deal with these sometimes hard realities is before a lethal confrontation, not after.

We cannot answer the question for our readers. Each one must answer it for himself or herself. Those with a deep moral objection to taking another's life may believe it is better to die, or for one's family to be raped or savaged, than to kill an assailant. We intend no condemnation of such principled people, nor would we try to dissuade them. They certainly should never keep a gun for self-protection.

But we believe that most of our readers would choose life rather than death, the ability to walk rather than a wheelchair. As terrible as it is to have to shoot someone, it is far worse to be shot or raped or crippled by a violent criminal. Victims who survive such vicious assaults are never the same. Psychological trauma can split families apart in the aftermath. Guilt, shame, and nagging fear are often the permanent psychological scars of being severely beaten or raped in one's own home.

The father and mother bear the primary responsibility of watching over and protecting their children. The have a natural duty to do their best to protect their loves ones. The unthinkable does occur to normal people every day in our country. The decision to recognize and prepare for criminal threats against one's family should be made individually after careful consideration. Children usually adopt their parents' attitudes toward important things in life. Showing them the value of preparedness and of learning to protect one's family is an heirloom, a gift of knowledge that parents can hand down through the generations.

For most of us, the will to live is stronger than the aversion to killing a predator. If you have thought long and hard, and have answered the Question in the affirmative, then you are ready to learn how to use a firearm in defense of your own life and the precious lives you are responsible for. The next chapters are a guide to these skills.

Endnotes

1. http://www.foxnews.com/story/0,2933,168509,00.html.

2. Personal communication to both authors by email, April 21, 2006.

3. Cicero: *Selected Political Speeches* (translated by Michael Grant), Penguin Classics 1969: 222.

4. Locke J *Two Treatises of Government* (Special Edition), The Classics of Liberty Library, Division of Gryphon Editions, New York 1992: 327.

5. Ayoob M. *In the Gravest Extreme: The Role of the Firearm in Personal Protection*, Police Bookshelf, Concord, N.H. 1980: 10.

6. Grossman D. *On Killing: The Psychological Cost of Learning to Kill in War and Society,* Little, Brown and Co., Boston, New York, and London 1996: xxix.

Chapter Nine

Tactics for Self-Defense

In this chapter we will discuss the situations in which self-defense may be required and the tactics suitable to those situations.

Criminal Assault and Use of Lethal Force—A Brief Summary

Home Defense

Public Areas

Automobile Defense

Women and Firearms for Personal Defense

Concealed Carry Tactics

Our purpose is not to go into great detail, but to broadly define the common scenarios of self-defense and their requirements of the defender. Further training and hands-on experience are essential for a student to possess confidence in confronting lethal force encounters.

Criminal Assault and Use of Lethal Force— A Brief Summary

How can you prepare to win a violent encounter if it is thrust in your face? How can you win a violent encounter? What will you do if you are suddenly attacked by a crazed felon intent on killing you? How do you respond to your door being forced open in the middle of the night? What if a carjacker suddenly breaks your window and leaps inside with a weapon? When is it legal to shoot a criminal who is attacking you, your friends, or your family members? Most people have thought about these questions. But the answer is not as simple or as straightforward as it might seem.

The 911 Myth Most American citizens are fortunate enough to be included in a telephone system that allows rapid access to emergency help by simply dialing 911 on the phone. A trained dispatcher answers, ready to take details about our emergency and ideally able to send help quickly. The good news is that our law enforcement officers are among the best in the world. They risk their lives daily to make our communities safer by enforcing the laws. The bad news is that they can't get to our home or location as fast as they want to. A patrol car responding to an emergency can only go so fast on twisting roads to a location that might be 5 or 10 miles away. By the time the police get there, the criminal has often completed his crime and left the scene. Typically it is too late for police to prevent or even interrupt the assault on the victims. Often their role is limited to beginning an investigation and taking a report, assuming the victims are still alive to give it.

In a life-threatening attack, call 911 as soon as the situation allows. But in the 10 or 15 minutes before the rescuers arrive, how well you respond to the deadly attack will completely determine the outcome. We see regular news accounts of crimes committed during or after 911 calls. We even hear the 911 audiotapes played on radio or TV,

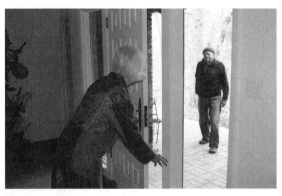

Tragically, even after calling 911, many criminals have already assaulted their victims and escaped the scene before police arrive.

with the frantic caller pleading for deliverance from a beating, a rape, or a shooting soon to take place.

Yet in spite of the horrifying inadequacy of the 911 emergency telephone system in preventing violent crime, many people amazingly rely on 911 as a talisman to ward off danger. Some politicians even promote the 911 system as a legitimate substitute for armed home defense, knowing that many people will believe the myth.

But a moment's honest reflection will make the truth clear—at least for the first minutes of a criminal assault, you and your family are on your own. The degree of injury and even whether you survive will largely depend upon your immediate and determined response, as you fall back on your training. In responding to most crimes, the police arrive in time to talk to witnesses and gather evidence for prosecution, assuming the perpetrator is even caught. As much as police officers wish otherwise, they rarely will be able to catch the criminal before he injures or kills you or members of your family.

Deep down, most people know the futility of relying on the 911 system to prevent crimes. Believing the 911 myth is simply an example of the denial that one's own family could be a target of violent criminals. As we have mentioned, overcoming denial is an essential step to making your family safe from violent crime.

Four Factors of Lethal Force Sworn police officers get extensive training in how to handle threats from criminal suspects. Unlike the average citizen, the trained officer of the law regularly gains experience in how to gauge and react to deadly threats. After any use of force, that officer's actions are put under a microscope as a matter of policy by his or her department, and usually by the media too. The officer must respond with a level of force appropriate to the threat, and no more.

Even more difficult, the officer must sometimes assess a threat and respond appropriately in split-second time frames, when the fear of imminent death is radically changing his or her perceptions. Tunnel vision, auditory exclusion, and tachypsychia (mentioned later in this chapter) are natural body reactions that anyone is likely to experience in a life-threatening situation. Juries must be carefully instructed in these realities and how they may explain an officer's actions that would otherwise look unjustified. These realities of how

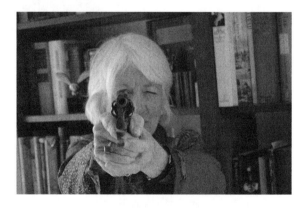

This is the only proven effective way to end a violent attack of a career criminal. The Four Factors of Lethal Force should be confidently known to all who choose to keep a gun for self-defense.

people react to deadly threats are unknown to the public and ignored by the drive-by media.

In a recent officer shooting in southern California a deputy was caught on videotape shooting a suspect. The grainy amateur film shows the deputy shooting the suspect, who was apparently responding to the deputy's agitated commands to "Get up, get up!" from a nearly prone position. Any lay person watching the video, which was endlessly played on television news, could confidently judge the deputy as guilty of an unjustified shooting.

But a jury quickly found the deputy innocent. They were able to see how he was in great fear for his life, that the two drunken perpetrators had shown extreme reckless endangerment by fleeing the deputy in a Corvette, going 100 miles per hour on city streets and finally wrecking the car. The deputy's defense team showed how the suspects had deliberately baited the deputy, challenging and menacing him even after he had detained them, alone on a deserted road with no backup immediately available.

Because the deputy's defense lawyers were able to put the jury in the deputy's shoes at the time of the shooting, they were able to see the deputy's actions as reasonable and justified. But, as is typical in these situations, the deputy still faces the second legal assault, this time on his family's financial security by way of a lawsuit.

An armed citizen gets no break for not being a professional when it comes to the law's judgment on his use of force. A citizen must know enough about the law of lethal force to be able to avoid or defend against charges of wrongful use of that force. The authors don't presume to teach fine points of the law. And as we have pointed out already, jurisdictions around the country vary in their application of a given legal principle.

But in general, four elements are required for an average citizen legally to use deadly force to stop an attack. These four factors must be present at the time the deadly force is used:

> *Ability*—The criminal must have the ability to harm you. For example, you must see that he has a gun, knife, screwdriver, or other weapon.

Opportunity—The criminal must be physically close enough to you to harm you with the weapon he has in hand.

Jeopardy—The criminal indicates by words or actions an intent to do harm that would make a reasonable person believe he was in imminent jeopardy of death or grave bodily harm.

Preclusion—No lesser degree of force would have worked in stopping the criminal from carrying out their violent act

The finer points of establishing your compliance with these requirements in a court of law is beyond the scope of this book. But you can be reasonably sure that you have met the legal prerequisites for using lethal force if these four conditions are present. The criminal must demonstrate to the prospective victim the *ability* to cause him harm, the *opportunity* to do so, and must have threatened the victim in a way that a reasonable person would believe his life or limb to be in *jeopardy* (or the life or limb of a family member or other person under his protection). Finally, the prospective victim should have *exhausted all other possibilities short of deadly force*. Such possibilities include running away, driving away, or closing the front door.

InSights Training Center, Inc. has described four guidelines for the lawful use of deadly force:

Drawing or using a weapon is justified only to protect the individual's life or the life of another innocent person, when no other means of defense would be effective. The armed defender should never display a weapon recklessly or use it in a needlessly menacing manner.

Although worst-case scenarios are a necessary part of self-defense training and evaluating tactical judgment, the armed defender should always try to avoid any situation that would require him or her to fire or even draw the weapon.

The safety of innocent persons is of paramount importance. Thus any person who believes that a lethal confrontation is imminent should first consider all safe alternatives to confrontation. These may include retreat, use of available cover, de-escalation skills, or calling for assistance.

Do not pursue a suspect. Trying to make a so-called citizen's arrest is in most cases not worth the risks involved. Police officers are trained and authorized to pursue suspects. Citizens are rarely obligated to do so. In almost every case a citizen defender should break off the fight and not pursue a suspect.

Defending against violence does not always require the use of violence. Some nonviolent methods may stop an aggressor—avoidance, talking your way out of a confrontation, or forcefully commanding the potential attacker to stay away. A simple display of power may make an attacker think twice about his choice of victim. This could be the prospect of police officers arriving, or the defender showing a confident posture and the ability to defend himself or herself.

Further along the force continuum are hands-on defense techniques, clubs or sticks, pepper spray, electric stun devices, knives, swords, guns, and other weapons. Each has its advantages and disadvantages. In this book we will focus mainly on the use of the firearm.

The most important tactical weapon is the brain. Mental conditioning is one of the highest priorities in learning self-defense combative techniques. The mindset of determination to fight and win is all-important. It is far more crucial to survival than the type of gun or the caliber of bullet you use. Many complex physiological changes occur in response to a deadly threat. A person fighting for his or her life often experiences tunnel vision, loss of acuity for near vision, auditory exclusion (not hearing noises or guns firing), sweaty palms, tachypsychia (the illusion of time slowing down), lapses in awareness, tachycardia (fast heart rate), and other "fight or flight" responses. These defense mechanisms can be perplexing and sometimes frightening. But if the student is aware of them, he or she can learn to expect them and effectively deal with them. Experts in self-defense have described a "combat mindset", a mental attitude necessary to surviving a deadly encounter. A student trained with the combat mindset knows these physiologic effects and uses them to his or her advantage.

Color Codes of Awareness Most readers are aware of the five-color coding system implemented by the Department of Homeland Security. This system employs five stages of readiness gauged to the corresponding level of terrorist threat. The stages are, from lowest to highest threat level, green, blue, yellow, orange, and red.

Training for criminal threat management uses a similar system, variations of which have been around since World War II. The five-level color code is keyed to the degree of mental awareness required to react to varying levels of personal threat in one's immediate environment. In general, as the index of suspicion about a potential criminal's behavior or perceived threat increases, the combative mindset should increase in alertness.

> *White*—completely unaware of surroundings; four-second reaction time at best
>
> *Yellow*—relaxed alertness; should be the minimum level of awareness when carrying a weapon; cautious, aware of surroundings
>
> *Orange*—specific alert to a source of potential danger; sense that something is not right; start to position yourself behind or near cover; be moving; consider legal ramifications, review the four factors justifying lethal force; mentally rehearse your actions and tactics should the fight begin; look 360 degrees around you, maintain global awareness, watch for accomplices or others sneaking up behind
>
> *Red*—The fight is imminent; employ de-escalation skills; attempt to retreat from source of danger; present firearm only if legally justified and mentally prepared to shoot; be ready to employ necessary actions if triggered; triggers would be any weapon produced; any weapon directed at you; aggressive movement by opponent
>
> *Black*—fight confirmed, opponent is attacking; retreat no longer a viable option; apply the force necessary to end the conflict

When the threat escalates to condition Black the fight is on. Use the acronym SAS, for <u>S</u>urprise, <u>A</u>ggressiveness, and <u>S</u>peed. Use ruthlessness to impart fear to your attacker. Fight like a bear, and if you are going to be a bear, be a grizzly.

When attacked, attack back, responding with unarmed or armed defense as the situation dictates. Do not let fear or anger control you. Instead, channel your anger or fear to your advantage in a controlled response designed to end the threat. Keep your actions tactically sound. When the threat ends, you must also stop your defensive attack.

After the Encounter

Soon after the violent encounter, police should arrive. When they arrive at the scene they will likely not know who you are. They will not know who the criminal is, nor the circumstances of the encounter other than someone may have fired shots. Police training dictates a cautious approach that allows the responding officers to gain control of a potentially deadly situation. Your proper actions will help them know that you are not a threat to them—you are the good guy.

1) Do not approach the police with a gun or weapon in your hand. Move slowly, clearly identify yourself, and show your hands at all times. Your hands should be empty unless you must cover a criminal assailant.

2) Listen to the police officer and obey all commands.

3) Comply with law enforcement directions. The police will likely ask you to lie on the ground with your hands out, palms up, and will handcuff you and others at the scene initially. After identification of all parties is confirmed and the police decide they will not arrest you, they will release you. If you approach the police with a gun in your hand, you may be shot. Even though you know that you are the good guy, the police would be perfectly justified in shooting you because you represented a threat to the officers. They have no way of knowing you are the victim until they do their own investigation. Sadly, some innocent victims have been shot by police officers because they inadvertently made moves that the officers considered threatening.

4) If you have shot someone, call for an ambulance as soon as possible, or ask witnesses to call for one. Most shootings

involve trials, and at these trials the 911 phone call is often introduced as evidence. The jury will hear a kind and compassionate citizen urgently requesting an ambulance for the injured criminal who moments before may have been trying to kill you and your family. Aside from being the humane and ethical thing to do, your request for medical help for the criminal who tried to kill you will make a powerful statement to a jury about the kind of person you are.

5) When the police arrive, tell them only the simple facts about the incident. You might say, "I was in my kitchen, he broke my door down, and I got my gun, went to protect my child in the crib, and told him to leave. He came closer with a knife, and I was afraid for my child's life and my life, and I couldn't run away, so I had to shoot him as he came closer. My gun is over there. Before I talk any more, I would like to talk to my lawyer." Or even more simply, "That man tried to kill my child and me. I know how serious this is, and I would like to speak with my lawyer."

Remember that immediately following a shooting, most people are extremely emotionally upset. Giving a coherent account is nearly impossible, and your recollection of events may be different when you have settled down emotionally and can think more clearly. Any discrepancy in your story may be used against you. In fact, anything you say can and will be used against you if the police decide to arrest you and if criminal charges are filed against you. At that point, the police are not your friends. You will need a skilled criminal defense lawyer to guide you through the adversarial procedures of our legal system.

It is better to comply with the officer's basic questions, and then to exercise your right to speak with your lawyer before any detailed questioning. It may be beneficial to conduct such an interview a day or two afterwards, when you can clearly communicate what happened. Your lawyer will know the best way to handle this situation and protect your rights. That's his or her job.

Post traumatic stress disorder (PTSD) is a very real and recurring problem for survivors of life-threatening altercations or fights ending in a death, even if everything was perfectly legal and properly done. Knowing what emotional reactions to expect from surviving a lethal encounter goes a long way toward dealing with these upsets and resolving them. This learning in advance is part of developing a combat mindset.

The almost inevitable civil lawsuit and trial are an emotional rollercoaster, a tremendous drain on mental and financial resources. Citizens who have lawfully killed another human being in self-defense are forever remembered for having done it, and many fellow citizens are uncomfortable being around them. In a biblical sense of moral judgment, they can be said to bear the mark of Cain, as undeserved as it may be. Social isolation, loss of friendships and careers, and long-term psychological devastation may follow, affecting the survivor and his whole family.

As with other life-dislocating traumas, supportive family and friends can help a survivor of a life-threatening assault regain peace of mind. Strong religious faith can provide powerful sustenance during recovery.

Good training in self-defense law is part of the process of becoming skilled in self-defense. We urge you to learn all you can in a reputable school about handling the aftermath of a shooting. This way you will survive not only the criminal's attack, but also the legal assault that will likely follow.

Home Defense

Most adults have wondered what they would do if suddenly awakened by the sound of the door being forced or a window breaking. This section will address the topic of home defense.

Perimeters of Home Defense American law takes the age-old view that a person's home is his or her castle. When designing a system to defend one's "castle", the homeowner should first determine what threats are most likely and the most dangerous. Is there a need to warn or protect children playing in the back yard? How great is the threat of home invasion or burglary? Do you want a burglar alarm system that works only when you are away on vacation? Do you want a warning system to activate each night while the family is sleeping? Could house pets accidentally trigger the burglar alarm? Should you buy a watchdog or guard dog?

As we have fire detectors to help us identify and react to a house fire, we can similarly develop systems to detect strangers approaching the house or entering silently or violently. The concept of perimeters is a convenient way to structure your defense. A would-be intruder is forced to deal with one or more outer perimeter detection or alarm systems, and then inside the home yet another layer of alarm systems and defenses.

The earliest warning provided by an outer perimeter could be vibration-sensitive motion detectors, infrared motion detectors, or video camera surveillance systems. Security guards and watchdogs provide a more sophisticated level of protection, although most of us cannot afford private security guards.

To begin constructing a layered home security system, look at your house, outbuildings, and surrounding land. With proper landscaping you can make it harder for criminals to hide on your property or approach undetected. Are there thick bushes next to the house that burglars can hide behind while trying to break in? Do you have nighttime outdoor lighting adequate to eliminate dark hiding places? Some burglaries occur at night, and a dark yard with an easy, undetectable approach makes a home a more likely target. Daytime burglaries are more frequent, and the homeowner should consider cutting down trees or bushes that hide the house from watchful neighbors. A house removed from a neighbor's eyesight by thick woods or a remote, rural location may benefit from a gate that blocks entrance of unwanted cars and strangers.

A reliable remote-controlled gate can be installed for less than $600. Friends and relatives can be given a simple password code that allows them easy entry. Remember that many burglars test a potential home to rob by simply driving up to the house and ringing the doorbell. If someone answers the door, the criminal can offer a simple excuse for being there, such as asking for directions in the neighborhood. But if nobody answers the door, then the burglar may enter the house with less risk of being caught.

An outside dog functions as both an alarm and a security guard. Some breeds have been selectively prepared for this job by careful breeding for physical and temperamental traits. Guard dogs are willing and able to inflict severe bodily harm on an intruder, and their effectiveness brings advantages and disadvantages.

An ideal guard dog would bark loudly at an approaching stranger, but would not bite the neighbors who stroll up to deliver a holiday gift. Guard dogs are not suitable for every home. Breeds vary widely in their aggressiveness toward strangers, from submissive to highly dangerous. If you do choose to have a guard dog, be sure you know the breed's behavioral characteristics first. Even a well-trained guard dog can occasionally pose a risk to neighbors or visiting children. This is an important decision, and many will choose to get their dog from a reputable breeder, who is more likely to provide you with a dog of stable and predictable temperament. Often a small-to-medium size mixed-breed dog from the local animal shelter can be a good guard dog, barking when anyone approaches the house, yet not biting anyone. Common sense and education go a long way in choosing the ideal dog to address this security issue.

In spite of any disadvantages guard dogs may pose, they are a highly valued resource in a home security system. Surveys of criminals in prisons show that a dog barking in a yard or inside the house will in most cases cause the criminal to leave and seek an easier house to rob. Criminals do not want to get caught, and they generally fear getting bitten by a dog. A barking dog is a loud warning to anyone within hearing range. As we discuss below in the section on burglar alarms, even a three-pound toy dog with a loud bark is a good early warning system for the homeowner.

If a criminal should get past the outer perimeter undetected, the next layer would be the outer building walls, windows, and doors. The simple habit of locking windows and doors will keep out all but the most determined crooks. The presence of people or barking dogs outside or inside the house will make most burglars go away and seek an easier house to burglarize.

Locking doors and windows prevents many crimes, since many burglars are simply opportunists. They walk by a house, ring the doorbell to see if anyone is home, and then simply walk around the outside of the house pulling on windows and turning doorknobs. Unlocked doors and windows allow easy, silent entry inside the house. They are an open invitation to a burglar. Most of us do not lock doors all the time, but the simple measure of locking up at night and when leaving the home is an effective method of securing the house's perimeter.

Still, it is important to realize that a determined criminal cannot be locked out. A simple crowbar will get an experienced burglar inside a house in about five seconds. A sliding glass window can be shattered in a second with a muffled rock or sharp metal object. Windows can be cut with a glasscutter and gently tapped to make a quiet and clean entry. Criminals have even used a chainsaw to cut through the side of a house or business to make a new doorway to enter the structure and remove valuables, or worse.

The lesson for the homeowner is that simple time-tested techniques of establishing external security perimeters will discourage most burglars. But no method can guarantee that a criminal will not be able to enter your home.

Burglar Alarms A burglar alarm system is the next layer of security. It is part of the inner perimeter system that can be activated by breaking glass, opened windows or doors, motion detectors, or walking on special sensors on the floor. The family members inside may press a panic button, causing an instant loud burglar alarm and perhaps automatically calling the security company who would urgently dispatch police to the home.

The value of a dog inside or outside the home cannot be overemphasized. These creatures truly are man's best friends, and a good family dog that barks at strangers and abnormal sounds in the house is worth its weight in gold.

Here we distinguish between the guard dog with the ability to attack and the watchdog, which can be either a big, menacing dog or a tiny lap dog. Big dogs cause more fear and hesitation on the burglar's part, but a small dog that barks at a burglar trying to jimmy the back door lock is quite effective in notifying the owner that something is wrong. People in rural areas may want a dog positioned in each of two layers of defense—one dog that lives and sleeps outside and another dog that stays mostly inside. Remember that any security system is more effective when it uses multiple layers of deterrents and protection.

Burglar alarms may be bought or rented, and may be self-installed or professionally installed. These systems may be stand-alone, or may integrate a telephone call-in home monitoring company. Phone systems may be battery-powered cell phone systems, or may simply make an automatic warning phone call to the security company on a regular land line. A vulnerability of the latter system is that many criminals will cut phone lines before breaking and entering a home or business. Homeowners should consider securing the phone-line entry wires by hiding them or encasing them in heavy steel pipes. A cell phone notification system avoids this vulnerability of land lines.

Another advantage of having an alarm company is that additional alarms can be installed in the same system—a fire alarm, water-flooding alarm, or freezer thawing alarm. The only disadvantages of these systems are the expense and the occasional false alarm. But the peace of mind that a good home alarm system brings is often worth the expense, especially when your family is away from home.

Safe Room What measures can you take if a criminal somehow gets pasts your external perimeter, then breaches a locked door or window and enters your home with family members inside? The next perimeter can be a locked bedroom door or other inside room that you have previously designated as a safe room. This is a specially prepared, secure room that all children and adults in the home would run to in the case of an unexpected intrusion. This safe room would ideally have a phone for calling 911. A mobile phone is preferable, since the intruder may have cut the land line. A well-known tactic of experienced burglars is to break into a home and immediately take one phone off the hook, thus disabling all other phones in the house. The safe room may have a shotgun, pistol, or other firearm stored safely for use by adult family members if and only if the criminals came crashing or shooting through the safe room door.

Homebuilders have become aware of the concept of safe rooms and can often construct one as an integral part of the home. Such rooms can be equipped with heavy security doors, bullet-proof cover, protected telephone lines or cell phone, gun safes or racks, and food and water provisions.

The Final Option Your firearm is the final perimeter of defense. If all other layers of warning or denial of entry failed, and the criminal is inside with you or family members, you are in grave danger. If you're lucky, the crook will at some point be deterred by the prospect of being recognized or caught and will simply leave. Burglars frequently commit crimes against persons in addition to stealing. Many serial rapists start their careers with simple home robbery, progressing over time to committing rape, mayhem, and murder in the homes they violate. Police in several countries now routinely collect DNA samples with simple mouth swabs from all burglars and other criminals to use as evidence in later investigations if needed. Samples go into a national database, allowing future matches with physical evidence collected in future criminal cases.

If you're unlucky, the criminal may actually want more than simply stealing your stereo or jewelry. He may intend to harm someone. You will not know his intent until the crime is completed and he runs out the door. Therefore you need to be prepared

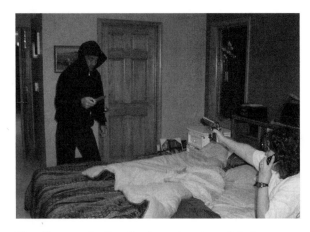

The firearm is the final perimeter of defense.

for any level of threat from the intruder, up to and including the threat of death or grave bodily harm.

What will you do when faced with a stranger who is empty-handed but approaching you? What will you do if he or she has a knife? Or a gun? What if the intruder is running away with your expensive jewelry box in hand? What is an appropriate response? You may have only a fraction of a second to decide. By falling back on your training you should be able to choose the correct response immediately and almost by reflex. You will rapidly consider many factors. Where are other family members? Is anyone in immediate danger? Is the criminal heading out the door or up the stairs toward a spouse or sleeping children? Is that a knife in his hand, or a screwdriver, or a gun? How close is the criminal? If he is 21 feet away, he can still run up to you and stab you in less than 2 seconds, likely before you can draw and shoot a firearm. Does the suspect have a gun? Can you draw and shoot before the criminal shoots you? If he doesn't know you're there, should you yell out a warning? Or should you shoot the suspect in the back before he can quickly spin and get a quick shot off at you in a microsecond? These questions are best discussed, learned, and addressed in the setting of a qualified firearms instruction school. Some answers may vary, depending on the mindset of the student. However, proper mental conditioning requires that these key decisions be thought out in advance.

The gun is a force equalizer. With it, and the knowledge to use it, a small, elderly woman can neutralize a criminal's violent threat.

The gun effectively makes her the equivalent of a large, dangerous man for the purpose of physically stopping a deadly attack. Similarly, if the perimeters of alarm and protection fail, a homeowner, father, mother, or other responsible citizen can use firearms to stop one or more criminals from inflicting violence on them.

In summary, the concept of layered perimeter zones is a practical and effective way for the homeowner to minimize the chance of criminal violence and successfully to resolve a violent encounter should it occur.

Public Areas

Too many people become victims of crime simply by being in the wrong place at the wrong time. Their chances of becoming a target of opportunity for a criminal are enhanced if they don't maintain an awareness of their surroundings.

As we write this chapter, a 19-year-old woman was reported kidnapped in a Midwestern state. She was wrongly taken against her will and is still missing. The last contact with her was while she was leaving her shopping mall job. She was talking on a cell phone to her boyfriend while walking across the parking lot to her car, very likely not paying attention to her surroundings. The phone line suddenly went dead, and she was apparently kidnapped. Unfortunately, criminal acts such as this are not rare. It is a nightmare for any family, and our prayers go out to the family of this young lady.

However, many of these situations are preventable. Most of us daily undertake potentially dangerous activities. Plugging in an electrical appliance, cooking on the stove, driving a car, and crossing the street all carry familiar hazards of serious injury or even death. Accordingly, most people pay close attention to safety at these times.

The danger may be less obvious when we are walking to and from our cars in a public place. Danger zones such as parking garages or lots may be located in densely populated areas, but still provide concealment for criminal activities. Kidnappings and violent crime usually do not occur in the middle of shopping malls with dozens of people walking nearby. But seasoned criminals are skilled at sizing up not only safe (for them) victims, but also safe settings in which to commit their crimes. Before starting the assault they try to be sure there are no witnesses.

Therefore, whenever you are alone, out of sight, and close to strangers, watch out. Use the color code system, and maintain at least an orange level of awareness. Watch the surroundings carefully and expect the unexpected. We do not mean to be paranoid or to be incapacitated by fear. We do advise being on the lookout for strange or abnormal persons or behavior. Talking on a cell phone or reading a book in this situation distracts you from your task of being aware of your surroundings.

Maintain a vigilant and confident appearance. Scan your surroundings. Make brief eye contact with anyone approaching letting that person know that you see him and are watching what they do. Do not stare, because that may be interpreted as an aggressive gesture. Don't look like food, or you will be eaten. Criminals will usually bypass any potential victim who looks as though he or she may fight back.

Watch for a second or even third stranger around you. This requires turning your head to glance in all directions occasionally. Be like an owl in keeping a 360 degree awareness of your surroundings, especially when there is a suspicious distraction of some type. Criminals frequently work in pairs or groups of three. One common tactic is for one criminal to approach the victim and initiate a conversation to draw the victim's attention, while an accomplice will walk up from behind, blocking an exit or striking the victim from behind unseen. If you see this situation developing, then shout commands such as "Stop! Stay back! I know what you're doing!" and get away fast. Be prepared to fight. Use whatever legal weapons or techniques are available, and win.

Avoid dark alleys, dark areas, or plainly open areas that are obstructed from public view. Get help from security staff or escort personnel when you have to walk through dangerous parking lots. Don't rely on security cameras to ensure your safety. Security cameras deter some crime and document it when it happens, but they do not prevent it. A criminal in a ski mask knows that in 15 seconds he can abduct a victim and get away clean without being identified.

Trust your instincts. They are a non-rational, emotion-based warning system programmed into your brain for a good reason. Do not ignore the suspicious gut feeling you get when a stranger does something unusual or spooky. Get away, create distance, be moving, and take necessary steps to prepare to defend yourself and your family. If the stranger persists, take appropriate steps. Voice your awareness of what they are doing and yell at them. This will often stop the attack, but not always.

If the stranger does something that signals an attack or violent motives, you should rapidly shift to condition red and immediately take action. In a loud command voice, yell "Stop right there!" hold your hand up confidently, and let the aggressor know you are aware of what he is up to. If the aggressor repeats back to you what you have just told him (e.g., "What? Stop right here? You want me to stop right here?") get ready for an attack. As we mentioned in Chapter 7, the aggressor repeating your command while he still advances toward you is the most reliable indicator that he is going to attack.

If he attacks, you are in condition black. You must instantly decide if you will submit or fight back with Surprise, Aggression, and Speed (SAS). If you think that all they want is your wallet or purse and nothing else, strongly consider simply giving it to him and escaping as fast as you can.

Too often, crime victims were not prepared with knowledge and skills to detect and prevent criminal assault. Perhaps they were not watching, were too trusting of mall security and cameras, didn't get escort help, didn't avoid hidden areas of the parking lot, became distracted, didn't trust their instincts, and didn't recognize a dangerous situation until it was too late. When the moment came, perhaps they didn't fight back.

In preparing to avoid such a terrible situation, you must learn and hone a defensive mindset that will allow you to win, whether the threat comes while you're in your car, walking on the street, or at home. Parents should take responsibility for educating themselves and their children about recognizing and avoiding dangerous situations. Gain the knowledge and skills that will enable you and your family to avoid criminal encounters, or to win them if they occur despite your efforts to avoid them.

Automobile Defense

Our mobile society requires many of us to spend considerable time behind the wheel of an automobile. Circumstances may require us occasionally to drive or even live in high-crime areas of town. Rarely a criminal may strike even in a seemingly safe suburban area.

Using firearms for self-defense in or near a vehicle requires a unique set of tactical skills. In this book we are able to cover this specialized subject only in a general way. As in other areas, your decision regarding whether to learn these skills is a personal one. You should make it after considering factors such as security threats, local firearm laws, and others who may frequently ride in the car with you.

Under the concealed carry laws of most states, if the driver or passenger is legally licensed to carry a concealed weapon, that person may carry a handgun on their person or stored in the car for ready access, usually out of sight. Remember that the use of a lap and shoulder seatbelt will restrict movement. Your choice of holster or concealment location in the car must take this into account. You should practice drawing while seated in your car with seat belts in place. As always, know the laws of the state you live in and any you may travel through. It is your responsibility to learn and obey firearms laws.

Awareness and prevention are the key words in traveling. Be aware of your environment and the threats it may contain, especially when going to an unknown area. Do not drive into bad sections of town unless absolutely required to. Avoid being blindsided at stoplights by looking in all directions while you are stopped. If you sense a threat approaching your car, drive rapidly away and avoid danger. If you have to, run through red lights to get away if you are fairly confident you will not cause an accident. Being ticketed for running a red light beats being mugged or worse any day.

Watch the movement of other cars in your area. A common tactic is for criminals in three cars to surround and box in the victim's car against a curb or building. With the victim immobilized and trapped in his or her car, the robbery or other crime is committed. If you find yourself in this trap, consider ramming through the blockade to get away. Your car can be used legitimately and effectively as a deadly weapon in some circumstances. Always watch for carjackers. Have a plan in mind for the scenario of a criminal running up to your car door and making demands. No car is worth dying over, and if you are by yourself and the carjacker demands that you get out and leave the keys, then obey if you think that is all they want.

Do not allow yourself to be taken hostage. If you are the sole victim, take the earliest opportunity to get away. Jumping out of a car going 25 miles per hour is very survivable. Being abducted to a secluded lot by a couple of carjackers is not. If family members or friends are in the car, especially children, you will not want to simply give up and let the criminal drive off with them still inside. Have a plan, know what is legally allowed, and have the training and skills to execute a proper response, whether it is a club, pepper spray, knife, firearm, or other means.

Do not pick up hitchhikers. You cannot know if the person you allow into your car is a poor student or an escapee from prison. The reward for your kindness may be an early grave.

Teach your spouse and children what to do if their car should break down. Accept help only from authorized car repair or tow company personnel or from people you know. If suspicious persons stop to help and your instinct warns you something is wrong, tell them to stay away. You can call 911 for a tow truck, at the same time requesting emergency police assistance. If they insist or behave aggressively, then get away or defend yourself appropriately.

You can prepare for roadside breakdowns by buying a membership in AAA, an affiliation of state or local automobile clubs that provide for roadside service. A mobile phone has become a must-have item for car travel. If you cannot afford one, you might be able to get an older mobile phone donated from your phone company or a women's shelter. In most cases, even if the monthly service has been cancelled, these older phones are universally able to call 911 when hooked up to a car battery with a 12-volt outlet cord. Each family member's car should be equipped with a mobile phone powered by batteries or a car's 12-volt cigarette lighter outlet. Remember that calling 911 is not the complete answer; it is only a part of solving the problem. A 15 minute response time from police or the tow truck is a long time if you are being attacked. The police will arrive to pick up the pieces and serve justice as well as they can.

The same laws of self-defense apply whether you are in your car or not. You should not risk your life in an attempt to protect material goods. If a criminal simply wants the TV or the car, let him have it and be happy to get away with your life. But if you suspect that the criminal has ulterior motives such as kidnapping, rape, or murder, then your life is in danger. A victim who doesn't fight back to prevent being abducted in his or her own car is much less likely to survive than one who fights back and avoids abduction.

The law allows you to protect yourself with reasonable means, and the use of firearms to resolve the conflict may be a reasonable response. When you shoot a criminal, the purpose is not to kill him or her. The firearm is a tool with which you stop the attack. As soon as you perceive the deadly threat to have stopped, or as soon as the criminal breaks off his attack, you must not fire another shot.

Women and Firearms for Personal Defense

Women are more vulnerable to crime than men for obvious reasons. Their smaller size and lower proportion of muscle to body weight make them much less able to fight off a male attacker without a weapon. Criminals, being mostly cowards, take full advantage of this disparity, preferring females as victims for their assaults, spousal abuse, rapes, and other horrific acts. The chance of a women being raped in her lifetime is 1 in 11. But like men, women too can take steps to avoid becoming a victim.

First, women should become educated about crime and the types of tricks and tactics that criminals use to victimize others. Second, they should learn always to maintain a high degree of alertness and awareness of their surroundings. If a trip to the parking lot or down the street seems too risky to make alone, a woman should get an escort. Third, women who wish to avoid becoming a victim should seek and complete realistic, practical self-defense training in unarmed and perhaps armed techniques.

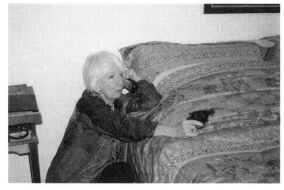

Remember rule three. Put your finger on the trigger only after making the decision to shoot.

Our women readers have likely seen many magazine articles about self-defense over the years. What is the best way to fend off an attacker? How does a woman protect her children and her home when the spouse or significant other is away? How does a 120-pound woman stop the brutal attack of a 200-pound male criminal?

The answer is in some people's eyes debatable and controversial. The authors believe that those who condemn armed self-defense for women are, to be polite, not being realistic. We strongly believe that the only sure way for a woman to stop a deadly attacker is to use a firearm as an equalizer and to shoot in self-defense if the situation is serious enough to warrant deadly force.

The book *In the Gravest Extreme* by Massad F. Ayoob (see list of recommended reading) is possibly the best discussion of the role of the firearm in personal protection. Ayoob writes about women's needs for self-defense, especially their need for a gun to have any hope of fending off a typical violent attack. He points out that hatpins, whistles, screaming, pepper spray, steak knives, kicking groins, jabbing eyes, and even karate are not only unreliable for self defense, they sometimes lead to even more vicious assaults.

Many women's magazine pseudo-experts recommend such pitifully inadequate techniques, and too often they end the article with the anti-gun statement "but police advise women not to get or use a gun." Ayoob, a trainer of innumerable police officers and himself formerly a sworn police officer, summarizes these non-firearm defense techniques in his own blunt but honest way. We quote him directly (page 38): "It's bullshit, all bullshit. Guns are the only weapons that put a physically small or weak person at parity with a powerful, very possibly armed, criminal."

It is true that people in our culture view it as highly unnatural for a woman to shoot someone. A woman considering the weighty issues of self-defense should consider her own values and answer the Question for herself. If, after becoming familiar with the realities of victimization of women, she thinks she is still not able to shoot a criminal with deadly intent, then that woman should not keep a gun for defense. Criminals can tell when a person is bluffing with a firearm, and they will very likely take the gun away from a person, particularly a woman, who does not show clearly her determination to shoot the criminal. This may result in the criminal using your own gun against you, a potentially worse situation than you started with. Unless you have determined beforehand that in deadly encounters you can and will pull the trigger, don't keep a gun for self-defense.

Women actually learn firearms training faster than men, and many become very accomplished shooters. The method of choosing a weapon for women is the same as choosing a weapon for a man—choose the gun appropriate for its intended use, of the highest quality affordable, and the most powerful caliber that can be handled safely and accurately.

The ideal caliber and type of gun is debatable. Some experts deride the small .22 rimfire or .25 auto pistols as "mouse guns," while others remind us that the first rule of a gunfight is to have a gun. If a person does not have the gun with them or easily available at the time of need, or if the person cannot shoot the gun reliably and hit the target, all the firearm training in the world will not help them. A woman should explore the choices and recommendations of those she trusts, get proper training, and then test-fire a variety of guns. She should choose her personal preference, ideally the most powerful firearm that she can shoot routinely without flinching or being afraid of its recoil. This firearm will have the greatest knockdown power that is practical for that person and will thus maximize her chance of winning a lethal encounter. As the legendary Texas lawman Bill Jordan said, there is no second place winner in a gunfight.

Some women are quite capable of shooting 9 mm. semiautomatics, .357 Magnum revolvers, or even larger handguns. Other women will find these guns too much to control comfortably, but will easily hit the bull's eye all day with a .22 rimfire pistol or .380 auto.

Many women find that a revolver makes a good self-defense weapon. One good choice is a comfortable medium-sized .357 Magnum revolver. This gun has the flexibility of shooting either .357 or .38 Special ammunition, both of which come in variety of loads, from mild to powerful. The recoil from a .38 special is quite manageable for most women, and this caliber still has acceptable stopping power. Women who are more comfortable with a stronger kick and louder muzzle blast can shoot the more powerful .357 Magnum loads in this same revolver, yet also be able to shoot .38 Special loads when target shooting or plinking cans around at the shooting range.

But in a lethal encounter one well-placed .38 Special bullet propelled by a modest powder load is worth infinitely more than six hot .357 Magnum rounds that miss the criminal. The most important determinant of stopping power is not how big the gun or cartridge is; it is shot placement.

Some women prefer a choice of several firearms. For example, many like the idea of a .22 rimfire pistol for practice and fun plinking and a larger pistol for serious self-defense. The ammunition cost is considerable, but not unreasonable. A box of .22 rimfire ammunitions costs about a dollar for 50 rounds. A box of 50 good-quality 9 mm. hollow point defensive ammunition will cost $12 to $16. Since routine practice is important, the lower priced .22 ammunition may make more sense for many of your trips to the range for practice. But realistic practice with the full-size pistol is equally important.

A rifle or shotgun may also be used for home defense, although the rifle's utility is limited by its tendency to overpenetrate. The 20-gauge shotgun has good stopping power and is manageable by even petite women. The 12-gauge shotgun kicks considerably more, but in semiautomatic configurations has a lot less recoil than a pump action, double barrel, or single shot design. Rifles come in many calibers, and most of these have a tolerable recoil that allows most women to shoot easily. Just remember that most rifle rounds of even modest power will easily penetrate through walls, doors, and other building materials to damage property, cause unintended injury, or even cause death.

Concealed Carry Tactics

Thirty-six states now have "shall issue" laws. These laws require authorities to issue to mentally competent, law-abiding applicants a license to carry a concealed firearm for self-protection. The spectacular success of these laws over the last two decades has been undeniable. The violent crime rate has dropped dramatically in those states adopting shall issue laws. Today there is little serious debate about whether such laws increase public safety. The reason is obvious. Even though no more than 5% of the population go to the trouble of becoming licensed to carry, criminals cannot tell who does and who does not carry. This uncertainty makes their work far more hazardous for them. Research shows that criminals shift their focus to theft and other non-confrontational crimes to minimize their chances of getting shot. The deterrent effect of shall issue concealed carry laws has lowered the rates of murder, rape, and assault in state after state.

Manufacturers of firearms and accessories have responded to the right-to-carry revolution with many new products—concealable handguns that pack a punch, specially designed civilian defensive ammunition, concealment gear, aftermarket sights, grips, and other aids. Firearm trainers have risen to meet the demand for training in concealment techniques, lethal force law, and tactics. Many states prescribe such training as part of the requirements for obtaining a carry license.

Tactics for concealed carry all have a similar purpose. The goal is to hide a handgun on or near the body, so that a casual glance from an average person gives no clue that a person is armed. The handgun is typically hidden in a well-fitted holster on the belt, under the shoulder, on the ankle, in a purse, or other location. This hidden weapon location should allow rapid access if needed in the event of a threat to life or limb. The key to successful concealment is a balance between the need for rapid access and hiding the gun well enough that it is not noticed. Methods of concealed carry are numerous, and a detailed treatment of their benefits and disadvantages is the subject of a formal concealed carry course.

Several factors will influence your choice of firearm and concealment method. You must consider how many hours of the day you will carry the handgun. Carrying a full-sized semiautomatic pistol all day can become surprisingly burdensome. You should consider when the threat is likely to be greatest and what position you will be in at times of higher threat (e.g., standing behind a counter, sitting in car, or walking down a street). In addition to a concealed handgun and spare ammunition, a plainclothes police officer may choose or be required to carry a flashlight, pepper spray, and handcuffs.

Hot climates pose more challenges to concealment, since light clothing offers fewer places for hiding your gun on your person. Remember too that state or local laws may limit or prescribe how a gun may be legally concealed. For this reason as well as variations in state laws on lethal force, we recommend taking a concealed carry course in your own state if it is available.

Concealed carry weapon (CCW) permits come with a significant duty to avoid fights whenever possible. Far from making the armed license holder cocky, the license should instill an attitude of sober restraint. Follow-up crime statistics show that almost all licensees probably already have this attitude, since their violent crime rate is consistently lower than the average population. It becomes even more necessary to walk away from such annoying but non-lethal harassments as insults. You must remain above such petty torments if you are to retain the appearance of complete innocence. The ability to convince a district attorney or jury of your absolute innocence is vital to your defense if insults escalate into a lethal assault and you have to use your gun.

Wrestling or fist fighting with a hidden gun strapped on your belt makes you vulnerable to your gun being grabbed by your assailant, with predictably dire consequences. With the power of a concealed carry license comes the commensurate responsibility to know and respect the law under which it is issued. Many businesses, hospitals, and churches do not allow concealed carry on their premises. The effect of such well-intentioned policies is, of course, to proclaim these areas safe for criminals, since only you and other conscientious license holders will obey them. Still, licensees who ignore these restrictions are subject to prosecution.

With all the restrictions and burdens that come with concealed carry permits, why even bother to get one? Since only a small proportion of the population (fewer than 5%) apply for and receive a permit, some apparently don't consider it worth the trouble.

Those who do go to the trouble of getting a license surely treasure the personal satisfaction and sense of security that come with being able to carry a concealed weapon. They may have experienced the terror of a robbery or assault and vowed never to be a victim again. Such a person has very likely looked soberly at the realities of life that many of us prefer to turn away from, and has made a rational decision to meet the challenge with a realistic and effective plan. More power to such a brave and honest person.

Each state handles the licensing process differently. After you fill out an application and pay a fee, your licensing law enforcement agency will conduct a criminal background check. A mandatory training course and passing of a minimal qualifications standard are required by most states. Typical laws require renewal of the license every one to four years, sometimes with a requirement to repeat the training course and qualification on the firing range.

Obtaining a concealed carry license does not end the need for continuing training. Routine practice, and an occasional tactics and combat pistol shooting course will maintain and sharpen your skills. If your legally required training course leaves you in doubt about your state's lethal force laws, get training from private training schools.

As one state after another has enacted its own concealed carry law, many have made mutual agreements to honor each other's laws. For example, the web site of the Arizona Department of Public Safety states:

> Arizona recognizes all other states valid permits: This state and any political subdivision of this state shall recognize a concealed weapon, firearm or handgun permit or license that is issued by another state or a political subdivision of another state if both:
>
> 1. The permit or license is recognized as valid in the issuing state.
>
> 2. The permit or license holder is all of the following:
>
>   (a) Not a resident of this state.
>
>   (b) Legally present in this state.
>
>   (c) Not legally prohibited from possessing a firearm in this state.
>
> (http://www.azdps.gov/ccw/reciprocity/default.asp)

The particulars of these so-called reciprocity laws when compounded by the number of states involved can be quite confusing. To make matters even more complicated, the laws frequently change, generally in the direction of more freedom to carry.

To simplify legal concealed carry for interstate travelers, Congress is considering a federal reciprocity law. Until such a law is in effect, we advise license holders to check the concealed carry laws of each state you plan to travel through, in particular any reciprocity agreements they may have. This task is made much easier by web sites maintained by issuing authorities, such as the Arizona DPS web site. The NRA web site www.nra.org also lists current reciprocity information.

Because the laws are complicated and change frequently, and because the authors are not qualified to give legal advice, we caution you once again that in no part of this book are we advising you on the law. If you have any doubts about whether your intended interstate carry is legal, consult an attorney with expertise in firearm law.

Be aware that some people may feel threatened by the idea that you are carrying a concealed weapon. Such fear is rooted in ignorance, but it can still make for some embarrassing moments. If such a person becomes aware that you are carrying, either through your accidental display of the weapon or otherwise, he or she may quietly call the police to report a "threat." You may be required to explain yourself to a responding officer.

Remember too that undercover law enforcement officers are typically quite expert at reading people. They may detect the subtle bulge or suspicious fanny pack that suggests a concealed gun. Even if your gun doesn't "print" through your clothing, an unconscious habit of patting the gun or adjusting it frequently can tip off an observant cop that you are carrying. If approached by a police officer and questioned, the permit holder should not make any fast or suspicious moves. He or she should show the officer their CCW permit and possibly the gun only after they show proper identification. All movements to remove wallets and firearms should be done slowly, and under the direction of the law enforcement officer. After all, the officer does not know if you are a criminal, terrorist, or just a regular citizen. He or she may shoot you on seeing your gun and any rapid, suspicious movement on your part. Common sense, listening to commands, and complying with slow movements should make the encounter benign and preserve your health.

In those states that have adopted it, concealed carry legislation has brought peace of mind and safer communities for nearly everyone. Whether to obtain a concealed carry license is a personal decision that one should make only after thorough education in the pertinent law and after discussion with family and possibly friends. We have confidence in the morality and integrity of law-abiding men and women to use the power of armed self-defense only for the good. Apparently, most Americans feel the same way, since most states have now revised their laws to allow concealed carry.

Chapter Ten

First Aid for Gunshot Wounds and other Serious Injuries

As with any health matter, the ideal prescription for keeping your family safe is prevention. We have discussed prevention of burglary by hardening the home perimeter, prevention of attack by situational awareness, and prevention of harm to one's self or family through self defense tactics and weapons. But however careful a family is, the world is not perfect. Despite your best efforts, your family may be injured during a criminal attack. In this event lifesaving emergency medical care or first aid must rapidly and appropriately be given to the injured family member(s).

In this chapter we discuss the priorities of responding when a criminal has inflicted significant injury to a family member. Discussion will include the five steps of casualty care, a new mnemonic that lays out the priorities of first aid, and several techniques and essential medical care products that should be kept immediately available in case of injury. These techniques are easy to use, and they may save lives. Sometimes the prescription for keeping your family safe will necessitate active measures to stop bleeding, support airway and breathing, and rapidly transport the injury victim to a hospital. The techniques described are relevant in any situation where a severe injury occurs.

In the following theoretical scenario we will examine a plan for managing injuries resulting from a criminal attack in your home or on your property.

After resting at home quietly, family members drift off to bed. Unknown to them, a criminal has escaped from authorities and is in the neighborhood. Coming to the first house, he finds the door locked. He runs to the next house and the door opens easily as someone forgot to lock it. He trips over a chair and a light at the top of the stairs comes on. The criminal quickly hides in the living room, as the homeowner creeps down the stairs. The wife retrieves a firearm, a 20 gauge shotgun kept for just this type of emergency. This family, however, didn't plan well enough.

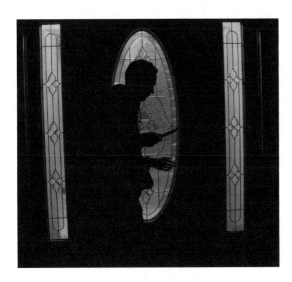

This attacker is now inside YOUR home... What is the most important step now?

The homeowner walks down the stairs with nothing in hand. Without warning, the criminal suddenly jumps up and stabs the man with a knife. After the struggle, the criminal runs upstairs to silence the rest of the family before they can call police. Without warning, a loud noise and sudden pain stop him. The shotgun blast to his chest has stopped him, and he falls down the stairs. He stirs briefly, and then lies motionless at the bottom of the stairs. The wife calls out for help.

What is the most important step now? The children awaken and come to their mother's side, frightened at what they see. *What should happen next?* The wife calls out her husband's name—only a moan. *What phone calls should be made? Are the children trained in how to call 911? What medical care should be provided, and to whom? Who will watch the children if she decides to go downstairs to see how her husband is doing? What if there is another criminal lurking downstairs? Where is the first aid kit, and what is in it that will make a difference in a knife stab or gunshot wound?*

The answers in this scenario are threefold. Some experts would argue that after calling 911 and requesting an ambulance and police, the children and spouse should remain in a protected location and wait for police. This line of reasoning acknowledges the possible existence of an accomplice still in the house who still poses a threat. House-clearing is dangerous work and is difficult to do properly even with two highly trained police officers. Others would argue that the husband is possibly severely injured and without medical care may die soon, therefore the armed spouse should quickly clear the nearby area and render first aid.

A third option is to call 911, and, knowing that the police may be 10 to 20 minutes away, consider calling a close neighbor who has firearms, inform him about the incident, and ask her or him to assist and watch for accomplices of the criminal. The armed neighbor would help provide security while the wife provides first aid to her injured husband.

In this chapter we lay out a plan of action that will increase the chance of surviving such an attack.

Five steps of trauma combat casualty care

Medical care for a victim of a gunshot or knife wound can be broken down into five steps.

The *first* step is to establish fire superiority. This means that you first must win the fight, using your tactical training and your gun. If a family member or friend is down on the floor with a severe injury, whoever caused it is likely not going to simply stop and give up. The criminal should be neutralized—either shot and disabled or held at gunpoint so he ceases to be an immediate threat to anyone. While this is being done, or immediately afterward, the defenders should be calling for help. This is the role of the 911 operator, who can dispatch both police and emergency medical support.

Remember that your 911 call is recorded, and choose your words with care. Later, in the calm of the district attorney's or plaintiff attorney's office when the recording of your desperate call is dissected in relentless detail, your words should convey the image of the good guy. First give the address where the attack occurred. Then ask for the police and ambulance. An audio record of your urgent request for an ambulance for the intruder you just shot will be powerful evidence of your good motives when you are called to account for your actions in court.

The *second* step is to minimize or abolish threats and prevent further casualties. This may include having police search and clear the house of further suspects. Further casualties or injuries should not occur if this is done correctly. If police are not there yet you can enlist a neighbor to watch your back or hold a suspect at gunpoint while you are performing other vital tasks.

The *third* step is to triage out the unsalvageable. This means that the family members, officers, or medical care providers should rapidly scan through all the downed or injured persons and identify those who are dead or have injuries incompatible with life. In the above scenario, the criminal suspect who has no movement or breathing and has suffered a traumatic cardiopulmonary arrest has less than one in a thousand chance of survival. When the phone call to 911 is made, the caller should describe what has happened, where, and who is injured. The dispatcher will send the needed emergency help, and for example, in the above case, would likely send police, ambulances, and other resources.

The *fourth* step is to move the surviving trauma victims rapidly to hard cover or concealment if necessary. If there is risk of further gunfire, the medical provider should carefully weigh the risks of exposing himself to it against the benefits of immediate medical care. Life-threatening injuries should be rapidly treated, and if there is penetrating trauma to the head, neck, chest, or torso, the patient should be immediately transported to a hospital or trauma center, (the fifth step). Injuries to the arms or legs with bleeding controlled by a tourniquet or bandage also require evaluation at a hospital. But with control of hemorrhage, such extremity injuries are not immediately life-threatening.

The *fifth* step is to transport the patient to more advanced medical care by ambulance to the nearest hospital equipped for trauma management. The best method of transportation will vary depending upon circumstances. Most commonly, an ambulance with emergency medical technicians (EMTs) or paramedics should be able to arrive within ten minutes and transport the injured to a hospital. If the ambulance, however, is going to be significantly delayed and the patient has penetrating trauma to the head or neck or torso, the patient will likely have a better chance for survival by being stabilized quickly on the scene, and then transported rapidly in an automobile or police squad car. Basic airway and breathing support can be continued in the back of a car. Bleeding should be controlled promptly as one of the first steps.

In summary, the five steps of providing care immediately after trauma are:

1. Establish fire superiority and call for help.

2. Minimize or abolish threats and prevent further casualties.

3. Triage out the unsalvageable.

4. Treat life-threatening injuries using cover and concealment.

5. Evacuate the victims to more advanced medical care.

Call A CAB and Go

The mnemonic **Call A CAB and Go** gives a quick mental prompt that takes you through the five steps in dealing with serious injuries.

Call for help—to eliminate threat, get medical care and ambulance.

Abolish threats—criminal, other criminals, prevent blood-borne pathogens, etc.

Circulation—control killer bleeds with local pressure or tourniquet.

Airway—make sure the victim has an open breathing passage.

Breathing—make sure the victim is breathing

Go—transport the trauma patient as soon as practically possible.

The first two elements, **Call** and **A,** deal with making the scene safer, and sometimes may be done simultaneously. You **call** for help from the experts while simultaneously neutralizing the threats. You communicate with family members and possibly neighbors to assist, and you definitely call 911 and have the operator get police and ambulance involved. You assist police officers in identifying the suspect(s), their weapons, the direction they may be traveling, and any other details that may help the investigation.

To **abolish** threats, the defender(s) will use force as needed to neutralize dangerous suspects. They will make the scene safer by returning immediate fire and dealing with existing threats (the assailant, other possible suspects, hidden weapons, etc.). This will help prevent unnecessary casualties. For gunshot injuries, a delay of thirty seconds spent stabilizing the scene will not make any difference in survival of the injured person. On the other hand, if a family member prematurely rushes to aid the victim, the gunman then has another target in his or her sights. Don't be a hero. Instead, immediately think "Call A CAB and Go".

The three letters **CAB** refer to emergency triage and medical care—maintaining the essential body functions of circulation, airway, and breathing. Triage means "to sort," and it is a dynamic process intended to prioritize the care of multiple injured victims. Rapidly assess each victim safely, which means starting with searching for weapons and disarming appropriately. If the family member is incoherent or confused from shock or lack of oxygen, he or she may shoot others in confusion, so always cautiously approach the injured family member and explain what you are doing. After the weapons threat is removed and with someone watching your back, assess and determine those who you can save and those you cannot. This process allows you to focus your efforts on those who can be saved.

Check carotid (neck) pulses and watch for breathing. If you don't feel a pulse, check the other side of the neck. If no pulse can be felt, you must make a choice rapidly. Remember that a trauma victim in full cardiopulmonary arrest (no pulse, no spontaneous breathing) has only a one chance in a thousand chance for survival. Don't do cardiopulmonary resuscitation (CPR) if there is a remaining risk of other criminals or threats. Move on and use your efforts to help those who may live.

When you have stabilized the scene, or moved to a point of relative safety, then begin medical care using the **CAB** approach for Circulation (compress killer bleeds with tourniquet or bandage), Airway, and Breathing. Note that this order of priority is different from that taught for civilian Emergency Medical Services (EMS) medics. They are taught "ABC" for airway first, then breathing, then circulation. However, in the acute combat trauma situation where the mechanism of injury is witnessed (e.g., you see a victim stabbed or shot), the airway and breathing are usually not a problem initially. Immediate control of bleeding has greater value.

C—Compress killer bleeds immediately with a tourniquet or compression battle dressing to maintain circulation. Note that 80% of preventable trauma deaths in combat environments are the result of uncontrolled bleeding from arm and leg injuries.

A—Make sure the unconscious person's airway (mouth, throat, and windpipe or trachea) is not blocked by the tongue or blood, especially if they are lying in the supine position (lying on the back).

B—Ensure that the injured person is breathing adequately, and provide rescue breathing as needed.

Go—As soon as possible, evacuate the victims to more advanced medical care. Planning is essential here. Things will go more smoothly if the whole family knows the location of the first aid kit, the basics of emergency care, and the options for transportation (wait for an ambulance versus loading into the family van). Penetrating trauma to the head, neck, or torso (back, chest, abdomen, pelvis) generally calls for an immediate "load and go" transport. These catastrophic injuries as a rule require emergency surgery in a hospital if the victim is to survive.

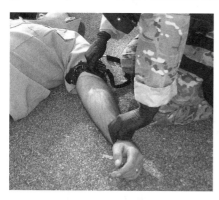

A tourniquet can stop life-threatening bleeding from penetrating wounds of the arm or leg.

In case of a stabbing or shooting wound to the arm or leg, a rescuer should rapidly apply a tourniquet and then later expose the site to ensure that the bleeding is stopped. If blood loss has not been excessive, then in most cases one should probably wait for an ambulance.

In the case of a "load and go" transport of a critically injured person, call the hospital en route. Giving the emergency department staff a quick heads-up phone call will greatly assist them in preparing for your arrival. If this is not done, gunshot and other major trauma victims arriving unannounced will always create confusion and result in less optimal medical care.

When you **Go**, know where to go and which roads to take to get there. Know which vehicle you will use, and what medical care can be provided along the way to the hospital. Having a plan relieves you of the added burden of making these decisions on the fly when your attention should be focused on saving lives.

If only one family member is hurt, and the criminal escaped or died at the scene, then caring for the injured person becomes a less complicated task. To ensure the safety of all family members, take the entire family with the wounded family member or make rapid arrangements for them to stay with the police or a trusted neighbor.

If a wounded criminal remains at the scene, an ambulance should be called while the homeowner keeps him steadily at gunpoint (finger *off* the trigger). If the criminal refuses to lie still and instead, without a weapon, stands up and walks away from the family and out the door, you may choose to simply let him go. It is important to not shoot to stop his escape unless you reasonably believe he still is an immediate threat to your family or close neighbors. Warning phone calls to neighbors are indicated, while you watch for new threats. Most criminals who break and enter into homes will operate in teams of two or three individuals, so watch out for others. It is likely that the weakened and bleeding criminal will be caught.

Remain wary of potential partner criminals nearby who may open fire on the house once they know that their friend is safely outside. Family members should ideally remain inside an inner safe room until the police have cleared the house and the surrounding area.

If after a violent encounter the violent criminal is the only one lying on the floor hurt, should a homeowner provide first aid?

A defensive shooting is a far different set of circumstances from, for example, a traffic accident. The criminal you just shot tried to kill or gravely injure you or your family. He made you use deadly force to stop him. This criminal should be considered a continued deadly threat until he has been properly handcuffed, searched, and rendered harmless by the experts at this task, the police. You do not know if the suspect is only lightly injured and feigning disability, waiting until you get close before bringing out a hidden knife or gun in a vicious attack. Unless you are a law enforcement officer who has been fully trained and equipped to neutralize injured criminal suspects, it is far better to stay back a safe distance and wait until the police arrive.

It is possible that you may have completely secured the scene, abolished any threats, medically stabilized any injured family members, and are holding the injured criminal at gunpoint, waiting for the police. If you are certain that all steps have been completed, and if you are equally certain that it will not compromise your safety in any way, you may consider tossing the injured criminal some bandages.

In summary, remember to keep the criminal covered with your firearm, watch for other threats, and make the family secure. When the police arrive be prepared to fully comply, to be disarmed, and to be handcuffed yourself (likely only briefly, once the police figure out what happened). Listen to the police, and do exactly what they tell you to do. Make no sudden moves, especially if you have a gun in your hand. The injured criminal will be taken care of by the police and ambulance crew after the scene is made safe and the criminal has been fully searched. Do not allow your spouse or neighbors to approach the victim in an attempt to provide first aid. If the criminal subsequently dies from his wounds while waiting for the ambulance, you are not responsible. He chose the course of action that put him in such dire straits, and you have no legal or moral obligation to risk your family's safety to save him from the consequences of his own evil deed.

With proper training, mental preparedness, and a well-developed combat mindset, the homeowner who pulls the trigger in self defense should fully realize the significance of that choice. If the suspect received no medical care because he posed a continued threat, that is a decision that you can live with. You have correctly judged that your life and the lives of your loved ones matter much more than this stranger who just invaded your home and threatened your family.

Some readers may think this approach callous, especially coming from authors who are physicians. But when faced with a potentially lethal threat, which is exactly what a wounded criminal suspect is, your first obligation is to save the lives of the innocent. Do not close the distance. Do not offer that criminal another chance to hurt you or your family. Wait for the experts.

If there are two or more victims on the scene when the ambulances arrive, the paramedics will likely triage the injured and care for the more severely injured person first. If one family member and one criminal suspect are injured equally severely, then make sure the police identify the family member to the paramedics. This person should likely be transported first, since he or she does not represent a physical threat to the ambulance crew, and therefore the overall care for 'both' of the victims will overall be faster. The criminal suspect will require a careful search by police for weapons and a police escort to the hospital before medical care can be provided. These necessary procedures will likely delay the criminal's treatment and transportation to some degree anyway. Treat first those first who are unlikely to hurt the healer.

Fortunately, the chance of a burglary or home invasion with injury to the family is small indeed. But we all know such disasters occur. The above discussion lists the priorities of providing basic medical care. Proper training, and re-familiarization and scenario-based training are essential. Providing that medical care well depends on having the necessary tools and supplies—in short, a first aid kit. We will now describe several key items that homeowners should include in this kit.

Essential first aid supplies for homeowners

A nearly limitless variety of medical supplies is available on the market. A fully prepared person could easily overdo it and stock a full sized room with enough medical gear to treat a small army. Any homeowner can construct a practical emergency medical kit fairly inexpensively that will allow him or her to help treat family and friends when needed, before the trip to a hospital. The medical kit should be sufficient for treating everyone in the family in a worst case scenario, such as a tornado or earthquake where there are traumatic injuries.

A comprehensive home medical kit should contain the following items:

(Note: the authors have no stock ownership or investment in any of the companies that produce these products and

receive no monetary incentive to recommend any particular products.)

Trauma bandages—2 for each family member. The authors feel that among the best is the OLAES bandage (size 4 inches), and also the Emergency Bandage™, also called the Israeli Battle Dressing. The Olaes ™ modular bandage (www.tacmedsolutions.com) is new and offers many features, including a gauze pad area that is packed with three meters of gauze that can be removed to pack a large wound. It also has an occlusive plastic sheet behind the dressing pad, which can be used for sucking chest wounds. It also has a pressure bar, and has Velcro ® control strips that prevent it from accidentally unraveling during the wrapping and application process.

Other choices in this category include the Blood Stopper Bandage ® and military bandages. Also remember that if a bandage is needed, a simple bed sheet or other linen, such as a cotton tee shirt can easily be used.

Tourniquet—2. Of the several types available, the Combat Application Tourniquet ™ (CAT) and the Special Operations Forces Tactical Tourniquet™ (SOFTT) are very worthwhile, and are the two officially used by the U.S. Army. Another easy-to-use tourniquet worth considering is the MAT™ (Mechanical Advantage Tourniquet). Many others exist, and all have their advantages and disadvantages.

Asherman Chest Seal (ACS ™)—2. This is a sterile occlusive dressing that is placed on a penetrating chest wound to prevent air from sucking into the chest, but still allows any high-pressure air to escape the chest. This decreases the chance for a life-threatening tension pneumothorax. Its one-way air valve allows air to escape from the chest cavity housing the lung, helping to keep the lung inflated and functioning. The seal comes with a gauze pad to wipe blood off the area so the seal will stick. There are other ways to accomplish the same goal, such as applying a one-way valve style dressing using a plastic occlusive sheet (*see* Olaes dressing above).

CPR mask with one-way valve and oral airways in case breathing support is needed. A small plastic oral airway set is also of value, varying from child to adult-size may also be used to prevent the tongue from blocking the throat, allowing the rescuer to give rescue breaths through the CPR mask. The oral airways and masks should be of appropriate sizes for children and adults. A range of 3 or 4 sizes should fit most people.

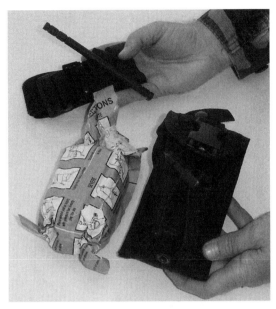

This tourniquet and trauma dressing come in a pouch. Consider getting one for the home and for each automobile. Train all family members in their use.

Kerlix 4 inch gauze roll—5. This wrap is used for wounds, abrasions, and light covering of burns. It can also be used to pack deep wounds if severe bleeding continues and a tourniquet cannot be placed, as in a groin or shoulder wound.

Large triangular cloth—for making an arm sling, applying a bandage, or head injury protection.

Large and small Band-Aids—for patching smaller cuts and abrasions.

Bacitracin or Polysporin ointment 30 gram tube—Apply to cuts, abrasions, and burns.

Liquid soap and several small brushes to cleanse wounds.

Rubbing alcohol (isopropyl alcohol)—for sterilizing instruments and cleansing skin.

Small and large scissors, scalpel, needles for treating splinters, minor medical ailments.

Small hand-held flashlight. Consider a small headlight with strap to free both hands.

Extra supplies of prescription medications for family members.

Over the counter common medicines—acetaminophen (Tylenol), ibuprofen (Advil, Motrin), antacid tablets (Tums), diphenhydramine (Benadryl), hydrocortisone cream (for poison ivy).

Other medicine: consider oral glucose in a tube for diabetics who may develop a low glucose level diabetic coma. Consider epinephrine auto injector (EpiPen ®) if any relative or neighbor has a severe allergy or history of anaphylactic shock from bee stings, certain foods, or medications such as penicillin.

Ace bandages, cold packs, simple splints—for orthopedic injuries such as ankle sprains. A simple 1 gallon zip-lock plastic bag can be filled with crushed ice and water for nearly all orthopedic injuries. Apply for 20 minutes, then off for 20 minutes, for the first few days.

Some other items may be added depending upon local conditions, special needs of the family, unique medical conditions, or other factors.

Home Emergency Medical Care for Gunshot and Knife Wounds

Triage—Who do you take care of first at a violent crime scene when faced with multiple injuries in multiple victims? How do you sort out, or triage, who gets treated first? The answer is broken down into three phases. You begin triage after you have called for help and have made the scene safe by abolishing any threats. Triage starts with stabilizing your own injuries, because you cannot help others if you are disabled by shock from blood loss.

Second, take care of your family and close friends. They are the ones under the umbrella of your protection, and it is your moral obligation to care for them as soon as you have ensured your own ability to function. There is also a practical interest in tending to your family members before any others. They are part of your home defense team. They may be required to assist authorities on the scene, manage a remaining threat, or assume some other vital task that another person at the scene may not be trusted with or capable of doing. You need your team members able to do their jobs.

Third, you examine and stabilize, as best you can, the others at the scene who are not dangerous. As discussed previously, if the downed injured person cannot be trusted or is the criminal suspect, then simply guard the suspect and wait for police to arrive. Take care of your own first, but rapidly progress to stabilize and care for as many other innocent victims as possible. Of these, stabilize the most critically injured first. Do the most good for the greatest number of people.

Penetrating extremity wounds and tourniquets—Consider what happens if you are involved in a gunfight and are shot in the upper thigh or arm, you see a lot of blood pooling on the ground under your feet, and you feel weak. After you neutralize the threat and hopefully have been able to call 911, you must act quickly to stop your bleeding. Should you apply direct pressure, or should you go for the tourniquet?

Experience in combat trauma situations has clarified the answer to this question—apply a tourniquet and do it fast. Many of those with gray hair have been taught not to use a tourniquet. That teaching has gone out of favor, and we have come full circle back to the old teaching. *Use a tourniquet to stop major bleeding as a first step, not as a last ditch effort. Do not try direct compression and then switch to a tourniquet after it has failed.* If you are injured yourself and choose to apply local pressure in an attempt to stop bleeding from a major vessel and this fails, you will eventually become weak and faint and unable to continue holding the pressure. Unless you have a partner to stop the killer bleed, you could very well die. One of the authors (EJW) has personally seen this happen in several unfortunate trauma victims brought to the emergency department.

We advise practicing applying a tourniquet until you can apply it with one hand, either left or right, to your arm or leg. The best method is to have one of the above tourniquets (CAT, SOFTT, MAT, etc) and use it promptly if needed. The next best answer is to use generally available articles for a tourniquet such as a one to two inch wide strip of material (nylon, clothing, trauma bandage straps, belt) and a small, straight stick or rod (known as a windlass) for twisting the material. Twist the material and make it tighten up around the arm or leg until the pulse or bleeding is gone, and lock it in place. Locking or securing the stick under one of the twists of fabric or some other way ensures that it will continue working in case you faint or move quickly from a danger zone.

Consider getting at least one for each family member, and train them to use it when the appropriate age is reached (usually about age 10 or 12 years old). Although a rope or shoelace could work, such a narrow ligature greatly increases the chances of permanent nerve damage.

How long can you leave a tourniquet in place? In operating rooms across the United States thousands of times each day, surgeons routinely apply tourniquets for several hours without any problems. Note the starting time of the tourniquet application, and if for some reason you haven't gotten to the hospital in one hour, then loosen the tourniquet briefly and test for bleeding. If there is bleeding, control it using local pressure only, but do not be afraid to reapply the tourniquet and leave it in place for another hour or two.

Management of minor and moderate cuts and gunshot wounds— Standard approaches to field treatment of minor bleeding have changed in recent years. An example is the scenario of applying pressure to a moderate wound, but blood is still oozing around the bandage. The old teaching was to simply leave the original bandage in place and apply new bandages on top of it.

The new teaching is that if firm pressure can't stop the bleeding, consider a tourniquet. If you want to try a second time to control bleeding with direct pressure, then apply strong pressure on the artery proximal (on the side closer to the heart) to the wound. Remove the old bandages, wipe away fresh blood and clots, and examine the wound. Then apply direct pressure with a new bandage exactly over the wound. If the wound has a large hole or missing tissue (such as from a high velocity gunshot wound), consider packing the cavity with gauze dressing and reapply firm pressure.

Gunshot wounds to the head and neck—These injuries tend to bleed profusely, and if the cranial vault that contains the brain is entered by the bullet, the injured person will likely be out of the fight, and often will die. However, much of the tissue in the head is not brain, and thus many injuries to the head, jaw, face, and neck are often survivable. If the carotid artery is struck, prompt application of firm direct pressure is needed. If the trachea (windpipe) is struck, the victim can often continue to breathe. But if the trachea is obstructed completely, the victim will be brain dead in six minutes from lack of oxygen. The only effective treatment here would be emergency placement of a surgical airway to allow breathing. This is an advanced medical skill that is beyond the scope of this book. The prepared family would consider local neighbors who may be medical professionals trained to do this, and would seek their help if needed.

Gunshot wounds to the chest, back, and abdomen (i.e., the torso), pelvis, or buttocks—A gunshot wound of the torso may result in death within minutes, or it may be survivable without any surgery. It all depends upon which part of the body is damaged. A gunshot wound to the heart is difficult to survive, even if the victim can be transported to the hospital in one minute. However, a gunshot wound to the lungs, abdomen, back, or pelvis is quite survivable provided that no major blood vessels are damaged resulting in massive hemorrhage. A one-way valve-type dressing such as the Asherman Chest Seal (ACS ™) or a plastic wrapper taped on three sides or kept in place with a loosely wrapped elastic bandage or trauma dressing makes a good bandage for penetrating chest trauma with an air leak.

For other torso locations, a simple bandage with mild pressure as needed and then rapid transportation are sufficient. The next step is for hospital personnel to get the victim to the operating room as soon as possible. A gunshot wound to the pelvis or major blood vessels of the abdomen and pelvis (the aorta, vena cava, or iliac vessels) may prove fatal within ten to thirty minutes. Time is of the essence, and rapid transportation is the key to survival of these serious wounds.

It is impossible to predict how badly the person is injured by simply looking at and examining the bullet entry wound. Bullets tend to bounce around off bones and other tissues. For example, a seemingly trivial gunshot wound to the buttock may travel upwards, bounce off the rib cage, and enter the heart, causing death within a few minutes. Therefore, any gunshot wound to the torso should be considered a life-threatening wound that will kill within minutes. Transportation to a hospital should be accomplished as soon as possible. A five to eight minute wait for an ambulance would probably be worthwhile. If the ambulance is likely to take any longer than that, it is usually better to place the victim in the front right seat of a car with the seat laid back, or in the back seat lying flat, and drive him or her to the hospital with no further delay. If possible someone should accompany the victim to provide basic medical care and attention to the ABCs (airway, breathing, circulation).

If you choose to drive the injured person yourself, don't forget to call 911 and the emergency room while driving to the hospital. You may be able to arrange an intercept with an ambulance, if the distance traveled or road conditions make that a useful option. In any case, you will be able to alert hospital emergency personnel of your impending arrival. Even a few minutes' warning gives the emergency trauma team valuable time to prepare and respond effectively to your arrival.

Training the Family in First Aid

Once a medical first aid kit is put together, the next logical step is assuring that family members have the skills to make the best use of it. The American Red Cross offers training in basic first aid, CPR, and use of the automatic external defibrillator (AED). These classes, available through your local American Red Cross chapter, are an excellent starting point. Those already familiar with first aid principles can update their skills to keep up with ever-changing protocols.

Although basic CPR training differs in minor respects from combat trauma care, it offers solid instruction in management of common household emergencies such as trauma, burns, choking, fainting, heart attacks and sudden death.

Beyond basic CPR, many excellent EMT and paramedic-level books are available. Basic EMT or higher level courses would be suitable for an older teenager or adult. Several shooting schools and academies teach emergency gunshot wound management (see Chapter 7). Some teach a mixture of basic to advanced firearm training and emergency medical care training. The internet and the local gun shop are good places to seek these advanced courses.

In summary, there is no substitute for preparedness. Maintain a first aid kit at home and also in each of the family cars. This will allow immediate and appropriate life-saving medical care response to almost any emergency. If a family member is injured by gunfire, the appropriate response could very well mean the difference between life and death. That response should follow the five steps of combat trauma care, summarized by the mnemonic "Call A CAB and Go." The goals are to stabilize the scene, patch up the wounds or apply a tourniquet, and rapidly transport the wounded to a medical center. Get the gear, get the training, and be prepared. Teach your family. The life they save could be yours.

Chapter Eleven

Learning Safety For Life

If you have progressed this far through this book, you have learned some sobering truths about the human condition. But you have also gained the uplifting knowledge that in a world where danger can intrude, your family can be strong and safe. You can make it so.

We authors have seen in our medical practices the effects of disease and injury. We have spent many long hours in emergency rooms cleaning up the human wreckage of violent crime. We have too often been frustrated in our inability to help the victims. In few other human affairs is the old wisdom more true: an ounce of prevention is worth a pound of cure. If our book can accomplish anything, we hope it will be to inform our readers that they have the authority and the power to keep violent crime from harming their families.

A firearm is but a tool, albeit a powerful one, to ensure a safe home. We believe that for most families the positive benefits of firearm ownership easily outweigh the negative aspects. Some readers will undoubtedly refrain from owning guns, and we fully respect that decision if it is based on fact, and not on misconceptions and prejudices. Some families should not keep firearms in their homes. Religious beliefs, the presence of unstable adults or children, or a history of spousal abuse or drug abuse may close off the option of armed self-defense. Still, the general principles of home security will be of some use to these people, even without the benefits of being armed.

Many families can use this powerful and beneficial tool—the firearm—to help bring their children to maturity, to enjoy sport through recreational or competitive target shooting and hunting, to cultivate camaraderie with others who are like-minded, and to preserve life. It can be considered a form of insurance, a final option to be used only in the extreme of mortal danger. Serious students of self-defense can rest better knowing that they possess greater than average knowledge and skills to protect their loves ones. They have learned the method of using a force equalizer to counter multiple threats simultaneously if need be, and come out the winner. They live in the world not in paranoia, but with relaxed alertness and 360 degree awareness that will detect criminal threats before they unfold. They raise their families and teach others to live with the same realistic awareness

Knowing that life-threatening confrontations are fortunately infrequent, the prudent owner of a firearm will still realize that regular, routine practice at a shooting range, perhaps simulating scenarios under pressure, is also a duty. The duty of a defender is to maintain those safe weapon-handling skills learned perhaps years before. He or she will as a matter of everyday routine store the weapon properly to keep it out of the searching hands of little ones. The defender will clean the gun properly, and maintain its proper functioning, because the jammed gun is as useless as a rock for self-defense. That person will teach others these duties and in the process teach respect, knowledge, and skill.

That conscientious defender will maintain proficiency in putting a bullet through the target, because the only shots that count are the ones that hit. That person will know that he or she cannot miss fast enough to win either an action shooting match or a lethal confrontation. The duty of the defender is to know the laws, to respect and abide by them. The duty is to accept as truth that unlike werewolves, violent criminals do exist, and that calling 911 will not save the family from their predations. The duty is to learn how to prevail in a deadly struggle and to endure as a whole family.

And after all, the skilled defender will know in his or her heart the satisfaction of fulfilling one of life's great imperatives—keeping the family safe from harm.

Suggested Reading

Ayoob, Massad F. We highly recommend three titles by this former police officer, trainer of police officers and civilians, and expert witness in the use of lethal force.

- *The Truth About Self-Protection.* New York: Bantam Books, 1983. Printed exclusively for The Police Bookshelf, this 417-page paperback is now out of print, but still available through Police Bookshelf. This sober introduction to the realities of self-defense retains the impact it had over two decades ago.

- *In The Gravest Extreme: The Role of the Firearm in Personal Protection.* Concord, New Hampshire: Police Bookshelf, 1980. A brief introduction to use-of-force law with particular reference to using a gun for self-defense.

- *Gun-Proof Your Children!* Concord, New Hampshire: Police Bookshelf, 1986. The best way to prevent accidental shootings in a home with children where firearms are kept.

Bird, Chris. *The Concealed Handgun Manual: How to Choose, Carry, and Shoot a Gun in Self Defense (2ⁿᵈ Ed.).* San Antonio, Texas: Privateer Publications, 2000. An avid handgun shooter and seasoned crime reporter, Bird draws on his wealth of experience to advise citizens on concealed carry.

Kenik, David. *Armed Response: A Comprehensive Guide to Using Firearms for Self-Defense.* Bellevue, Washington: Merril Press, 2005. A detailed review of not only the equipment, but the required skills and mindset of anyone who would own a gun for self protection.

Lott, Jr., John R. An economist by training and a prolific scholar in the field of guns and crime. We recommend these two titles.

- *More Guns, Less Crime: Understanding Crime and Gun-Control Laws (2ⁿᵈ Ed.).* Chicago and London: The University of Chicago Press, 2000. A classic exposition of how lawful use of guns for self-defense reduces violent crime.

- *The Bias Against Guns: Why Almost Everything You've Heard About Gun Control Is Wrong.* Washington, D.C.: Regnery Publishing, Inc., 2003. A thoroughly documented analysis of how media and scientific institutions are swayed by prejudice against guns and gun owners.

Malcolm, Joyce Lee. In these two books this historian and law professor writes authoritatively about the development of individual rights in America and Great Britain, especially the right to keep and bear arms.

- *To Keep and Bear Arms: The Origins of an Anglo-American Right.* Cambridge, Massachusetts and London, England: Harvard University Press, 1994. The author traces the right of firearms ownership as one of "those liberties secured by Englishmen and bequeathed to their American colonists."

- *Guns and Violence: The English Experience.* Cambridge, Mass. and London, England: Harvard University Press, 2002. Centuries of English history show Americans how *not* to formulate firearm policy.

Kleck, Gary. This professor of criminology has contributed much of what we know about the role of firearms in American society. Three of his books are recommended.

- *Point Blank: Guns and Violence in America.* New York: Aldine de Gruyter, 1991. An award-winning milestone in criminology scholarship, this book showed how often Americans use firearms for legitimate self defense against violent criminal attacks.

- *Targeting Guns: Firearms and Their Control.* New York: Aldine de Gruyter, 1997. In this follow up to *Point Blank*, Kleck updates the research, answers his critics, and documents the emotional reaction to his research among gun control supporters.

- (with Don B. Kates) *Armed: New Perspectives on Gun Control.* Amherst, New York: Prometheus Books, 2001. Kleck and constitutional law scholar Don B. Kates confront erroneous conventional wisdom about firearm violence with science-based evidence and historical fact.

Kopel, David B. *The Samurai, the Mountie, and the Cowboy: Should America Adopt the Gun Controls of Other Democracies?* Buffalo, New York: Prometheus Books, 1992. An early comparative historical analysis showing how America's tradition of liberty molded its gun laws.

Grossman, Dave. In two books Army Ranger and West Point professor Lt. Col. Dave Grossman, U.S. Army (ret.) cites military history in shedding light on the dark subject of the psychology and physiology of killing.

- *On Killing: The Psychological Cost of Learning to Kill in War and Society*. Boston, Massachusetts: Little, Brown and Company, 1995. The definitive modern text on the realities of mortal combat.

- (with Loren W. Christensen). *On Combat: The Psychology and Physiology of Deadly Combat in War and in Peace*. PPCT Research Publications, 2004. An exploration of how fighting for one's life affects the body and mind.